HEALING
THE
PHARMACY
OF THE
WORLD

An Inside Story of Medical Products Manufacturing and Regulation in India

I0391165

K.L. SHARMA

Formerly Joint Secretary, Drug & Food Regulation, Government of India

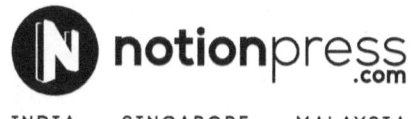

INDIA · SINGAPORE · MALAYSIA

Notion Press Media Pvt Ltd

No. 50, Chettiyar Agaram Main Road,
Vanagaram, Chennai, Tamil Nadu – 600 095

First Published by Notion Press 2021
Copyright © K.L. Sharma 2021
All Rights Reserved.

ISBN 978-1-63940-355-4

To my mother, eldest brother and bhabhi

CONTENTS

PREFACE

The Indian pharmaceutical industry continues to be an enigma. The mere mention of the sector is sufficient to evoke divergent responses from the stakeholders. Globally hailed as the messiah of low-cost medicines, the Indian pharmaceutical industry plays a dominant role in enhancing the global availability, accessibility and affordability of generic medicines. As the largest supplier of generic medicines at a fraction of the cost of innovator drugs, Indian pharmaceutical industry helps in improving the health outcomes and also impacts the health budgets in many countries. At the same time, it is ridiculed for the alleged non-compliance with good practices concerning manufacturing, clinical, laboratory, transportation, distribution and storage (GxPs) of medical products, as well as for data fudging and use of poor quality Active Pharmaceutical Ingredients. The poor-quality generic medicines, it is alleged, do more harm than good to the poor and further impoverish them.

Indian generics might have democratized and enhanced the global availability, accessibility and affordability of therapies; the allegations about its suspect quality, if true, pose serious questions of life and death. The differing perceptions about the role of the Indian pharmaceutical industry and its contribution to the cause of humanity continue to perplex many. It makes one wonder whether it is a real or a pseudo *messiah*.

I had the unique opportunity of having a ringside view of the governance in India while directly assisting Cabinet Secretaries, four of them, during 11 years in my capacity as Deputy Secretary to the Cabinet and later as Director and Joint Secretary in the Cabinet Secretariat, Rashtrapati Bhavan. This coincided with the last few months of the terms of Atal Bihari Vajpayee, two full terms of Dr. Manmohan Singh and the first few months of Narendra Modi's term as the Prime Minister of India.

During 2014 to 2017, I worked as a Joint Secretary in the Ministry of Health and Family Welfare (MoHFW) where, *inter alia*, drug regulation was a part of my charge. That stint provided me a lot of insight into the working of the medical products sector. The period witnessed a string of initiatives for reforming the medical products regulation in the country. These included amending the Drugs & Cosmetics Rules, 1945 and framing of the Medical Devices Rules, 2017. The drafts of the New Drugs and Clinical Trial Rules; the Sale of Drugs, including e-pharmacy Rules; and the Cosmetics Rules had also been prepared at that point of time. Prohibition of the irrational Fixed Dose Combinations (FDCs) in 2016, conduct of the largest-ever drug survey 2014–16 for determining the quality of drugs involving over 47,000 samples; conduct of risk-based inspections of a large number of pharmaceutical manufacturers and surprise inspection of wholesale distributors of pharmaceuticals in Delhi in June 2017 are the other few significant activities accomplished during that stint. The period also witnessed extensive collaboration with WHO and regulatory agencies of many countries for improving the quality of Indian medical products.

Having followed an open-door policy, I had the privilege of interacting with the most diverse set of individuals, medical practitioners, academicians, organizations, and consumer and industry associations in India and abroad.

After leaving the MoHFW in June 2017, I realized that the existing literature, findings of the regulators of countries importing medicines from India, observations, perceptions or complaints of whistle blowers and others cannot answer the riddle –whether India is a real or a pseudo *messiah* –with any degree of accuracy. I had a strong urge that the truth must be unveiled for the larger public good and I realized that it had to be done by a person who could contextualize differing perceptions to present a comprehensive and objective picture. After the onset of the COVID-19 pandemic, I could no longer prevent myself from thinking more and more on these lines, and that was the beginning of the present book.

Encapsulating the learning from the experience, this book traverses through the narrow confines of India's policy conundrum and in pursuit of the public good, unravels many hidden secrets. Like a karat meter, it looks beyond the surface and ascertains the true state of affairs of the pharmaceutical and medical devices sectors. The work presents a compelling context for the government and the Indian industry to wake up and take prompt, corrective and preventive action, *inter alia*, for leveraging the emerging geo-strategic environment that offers a second opportunity to the Indian industry in 2021.

The intricacy of public policy formulation and execution in a complex environment does not render itself liable to just one universal and optimal answer; it cannot be reduced to the binary of yes or no, good or bad. The book, it is expected, will honestly provide answers to the puzzle and clear doubts that had been lurking in the minds of many. It would be of interest to the central and the state governments in India; healthcare functionaries; professionals in pharmaceutical and medical device industry; Indian and global regulatory agencies; consumers, consumers/patient safety organizations, students of medicine, pharmaceutical sciences and medical technology; and the general readers who care for the quality of human healthcare.

The present work, however, does not have any pretensions to infallibility or being the panacea for all ills. This work is in pursuance of the dictum of Article 51A(h) of the Constitution of India that casts an obligation upon all citizens of India as part of their fundamental duty to develop the scientific temper, humanism and the spirit of inquiry and reform. Having made an effort to unveil the truth, I have discharged my obligation to the country and humanity at large; the choice to take it or ignore it is that of the stakeholders.

ACKNOWLEDGMENTS

I owe an enormous debt of gratitude to a number of organizations and individuals who have made it possible for me to bring this book out. To be fair, it is not just my work; it is rather the work of all those who have struggled painstakingly for decades to improve the quality of Indian medical products. As a conscientious citizen, I have only made an effort to bring together all the ideas that could help in disrupting the *status quo* and force transformational reforms in the pharmaceutical and medical devices sectors. It will be a great tribute to the untiring efforts of a whole lot of them if reflecting the true state of affairs of the Indian pharmaceutical and medical devices industry, which this work attempts to do, could break the inertia. As far as I am concerned, I am doing it as a part of a duty and an obligation that I owe to the country and humanity at large. In the process, I am sure I would have inadvertently and unintentionally disheveled some and also hurt the sentiments of a few others. The entire credit for the good work goes to the wonderful human beings, my seniors, colleagues and friends across the government, stakeholders from industry and consumer associations. The errors and omissions in the book are all mine.

First and foremost, I would like to acknowledge that but for the immense opportunities provided by the Government of India while nurturing me through four decades of my association with the government, I would have never ever have been able to comprehend public policy in general and the one concerning pharmaceuticals and medical devices sectors in particular. It was my privilege to have worked with, to be guided and nurtured by four former Cabinet Secretaries, Kamal Pande, B. K. Chaturvedi, K. M. Chandrasekhar and Ajit Kumar Seth. They not only trusted me but also encouraged and empowered me to be bold and decisive. This is amply reflected in the present work. Vijai Sharma, the former Secretary, Ministry of Environment, Forests and Climate Change, former Member of the National Green Tribunal and the former Chief Information Commissioner of India mentored and encouraged me during our close association in the Cabinet Secretariat. Many of my other colleagues in the Cabinet Secretariat, including those working in my team, helped me to learn the nuances of public policy. A number of other senior officials of the Government of India, present and former, helped in shaping my understanding of governance-related issues.

I was also fortunate to have worked with brilliant officers like Lov Verma, BP Sharma, R K Jain and CK Mishra in the MoHFW. They provided a lot of space to me to take appropriate initiatives to reform the medical products regulation. I must add that my association with KB Agarwal helped me in enhancing my patience. Dr. Jagdish Prasad, the then DGHS, also provided a lot of help when needed.

My colleagues from the CDSCO, Dr. V G Somani and Dr. S. Eswara Reddy, went out of their way to ensure successful completion of any task that was taken up. Dr. GN Singh, the then DCG(I) and Dr. RA Singh, Director, RDTL, Chandigarh were a great support and were always positive and helpful. A K Pradhan, Dr. Ravi Kant Sharma, Sanjeev Kumar, Rubina, Vishala, R. Chandrashekar and Arvind Kukreti from the CDSCO also played an important role in organizing a large number of stakeholder consultations. Rishi Kant Singh, Legal Adviser in the CDSCO was also always willing to shoulder additional responsibility.

I benefited a lot from my interaction with Dr. (Prof) B. Suresh, Pro-Chancellor, JSS Academy of Higher Education & Research and President, Pharmacy Council of India. Dr. (Prof) YK Gupta, President, AIIMS, Jodhpur and earlier a Professor and Head of the Department of Pharmacology in AIIMS, Delhi, and Dr. Surinder Singh, Vice-Chancellor, JSS Academy of Higher Education & Research and former Director, National Institute of Biologicals.

Dr. Jitendar Sharma, CEO, Andhra Med Tech Zone, provided useful inputs from time to time for regulation and promotion of the medical devices industry in the country. Late Dr. MK Bhan, former Secretary, Department of Biotechnology, Late Dr. (Prof) Ranjit Roy Chaudhury and Dr. Nilima Kshirsagar, Chair in Clinical Pharmacology, ICMR, Mumbai, volunteered to shoulder responsibility whenever they were approached.

Dr. Madhur Gupta from the WHO India office and Manisha Sridhar from the WHO, SEARO office made immense contribution in understanding the international perspective for improving the Indian medical products regulatory landscape. Karun Rishi of USA-India Chamber of Commerce continues his pursuit for enhancing India–US cooperation in the field of clinical research and clinical trials so that the Indian population can benefit from better medicines.

A number of associations of pharmaceutical companies and medical devices played a major role in visualizing a roadmap for the two sectors. Members of the Indian Pharmaceutical Alliance, Indian Drugs Manufacturers Association, Bulk Drug Manufacturers Association, FICCI, CII, ASSOCHAM and FOPE participated in large numbers in stakeholders' consultations for redefining the legal and regulatory landscape. Late DG Shah of the Indian Pharmaceutical Alliance, Pankaj Patel of Cadila Healthcare, Dilip S Shanghvi, Chairperson, Sunpharma, Satish Reddy of Dr. Reddy's laboratory, Kiran Mazumder-Shaw of BIOCON have all contributed in enhancing my understanding of the industry and the global perspective. Ashok Madan (IDMA), Anurag Khera (Glenmark), A H Khan (Sun Pharma), Vishwanath (Dr. Reddy's), Chetan Gupta (Emcure), Kuldeep (Lupin), Amit Srivastava (Johnson and Johnson), Dr. Ajay Sharma and Umang Chaturvedi made it a point to attend most of the deliberations in the MoHFW.

I must add that Rajiv Nath and his team from AiMED participated in all meetings and worked tirelessly to improve the medical devices regulatory landscape. From the medical devices industry, Probir Das, Pawan Chaudhary, Himanshu Baid, Gurmeet Chugh, Praveen Sharma, Sudha Mairpadi, Vaibhav Garg, Ashok Kumar, Sumati Randeo and Prabhat Jain volunteered and made significant contributions for evolving the policy framework. Bejon Misra, Founder of Partnership for Safe Medicines India was a key participant in many deliberations.

My PPS in the MoHFW, Government of India, Harish Jain, was a one-man army, taking care of all logistics and secretarial work. Hiten Sahu, *Senior* Consultant, CDSCO and Abhinav Kapoor, *Drug Inspector* worked day and night to complete the assigned work. NL Meena, former Member Secretary, Law Commission of India provided his services for legislative drafting. VP Bhardwaj, former Joint Secretary, Department of Financial Services also chipped in from time to time.

I must add that a frank interaction in a meeting with Dinesh Thakur at the behest of the Prime Minister's Office was very informative. I must, however, add that even before my interaction with him, I had gone through his representations to different Parliamentary Committees along with other complaints that had been received in the MoHFW with a view to ascertain the problematic areas and initiate corrective action.

I have also used the information, articles and documents available on the internet, including on the websites of the WHO, to the extent the relevant information could be captured from them. Since it has not been possible for me to acknowledge everyone individually, I thank all those whose names I have not been able to include here profusely for their unstinting support and guidance.

I acknowledge the hard work done by the team at Notion Press for giving shape to the book through their painstaking efforts.

Finally, I wish to thank my family members, especially my wife Geeta who left her job to take care of the family responsibilities single-handedly, both before and after my retirement from the government, and tolerated my incessant absence and permitted me to spend time for pursuing the work.

INTRODUCTION

RIGHT TO QUALITY HEALTHCARE PRODCUTS

The highest attainable standard of health includes access to safe, efficacious and quality essential medicines. Such access is an integral part of the right to health under the international law. The laws include the 1946 constitution of the World Health Organization[1] and 1948 Universal Declaration of Human Rights (UDHR).[2] The WHO Constitution, *inter alia*, recognizes health as a fundamental human right that is indispensable for availing other human rights. Article 25.1 of the UDHR defines health as a state of complete physical, mental and social well-being and not merely the absence of disease or infirmity. All women, men and others irrespective of their race, religion, political belief and economic or social conditions are entitled to the right to health and this right includes access to quality essential medicines.

The WHO document '*Ruling for Access- Leading court cases in developing countries on access to essential medicines as part of the fulfillment of the right to health*' elaborates the emerging legal position in different countries.[3] This document highlights that in accordance with the provisions of the Universal Declaration of Human Rights, everyone has the right to a standard of living adequate for the health and well-being of himself/herself and of his/her family, including food, clothing, housing, medical care and necessary social services. In furtherance of the search for a more grounded basis for enjoyment of human rights, two separate treaties *viz.* the International Covenant on Civil and Political Rights (ICCPR) and the International

---

[1.] Available at: https://www.who.int/governance/eb/who_constitution_en.pdf
[2.] Available at: https://www.un.org/en/about-us/universal-declaration-of-human-rights
[3.] https://www.who.int/medicines/areas/human_rights/Details_on_20_court_cases.pdf?ua=1

Covenant on Economic, Social and Cultural Rights (ICESCR) came into being in 1966.[4] The ICESCR, with over 160 states parties, recognizes the progressive realization of the right to health, subject only to the limitations arising from the availability of required resources. The core obligations under the ICESCR as clarified in Comment No.14 specifically include the access to essential medicines. These core obligations are not subject to progressive realization and each state party to the covenant is obligated to ensure immediate access to such medicines.

RIGHT TO HEALTH IN INDIA

India's commitment to international legal treaties and conventions binds it to provide a minimum standard of universal healthcare. Even though the right to health has specifically not been included as a fundamental right, Article 21 of the Indian Constitution guarantees the protection of life and personal liberty to everyone and not just the Indian citizens. Public health and the obligation of the state for provisioning healthcare also find multiple references in the Directive Principles of State Policy in Part IV of the Indian Constitution.

A Constitution Bench of the Supreme Court of India has held that the Fundamental Rights and the Directive Principles are two wheels of the chariot in establishing an egalitarian social order.[5] The apex court has also held that the Right to Life enshrined in Article 21 of the Indian Constitution means something more than mere survival or animal existence. It has read the right to health to be an integral part of the right to life and it encapsulates the provision of essential quality medicines.

The Supreme Court has further held that the Right to Life with human dignity derives its life breath from the Directive Principles of State Policy. No State, neither the central government nor any state government, has the right to take any action which will deprive a person of the enjoyment of

---

4. Available at: https://www.ohchr.org/en/professionalinterest/pages/ccpr.aspx
5. Minerva Mills Limited vs. Union of India [(1981 (1) SCR 206 = AIR 1980 SC 1789]

minimum requirements that must exist in order to enable a person to live with human dignity.[6] The combined reading of the Fundamental Rights and the Directive Principles of State policy, as interpreted by the Supreme Court, leaves no doubt about the obligation of the State to secure the right to essential medicines to everyone.

The above conclusions are cemented by some specific provisions in the Indian Constitution. These include Article 39 (e) which obligates the State to secure the health of workers, Article 42 relating to ensuring just and humane conditions of work and maternity relief and Article 47 making the State responsible to raise the nutrition levels and standard of living of the people and to improve public health. Panchayats and municipalities have also been mandated to strengthen the public health under Article 243G and Entry 23 of the Eleventh Schedule.

The availability of and access to quality medical products, especially essential medicines, is one of the key elements of good healthcare, and without the availability of quality medical products, it is not possible to lead a life befitting human dignity. Therefore, in India, it is a fundamental right of every individual to have access to quality essential medicines. Provisioning of quality medical products for improving the health conditions of the people, in this background, is therefore a fundamental obligation of the Indian State.

ACCESS TO AND AFFORDABILITY OF MEDICAL PRODUCTS

The quality, safety and efficacy/efficiency of medical products are critical for efficient healthcare delivery. In today's world, with a large number of debilitating diseases afflicting humanity, quality medicines and medical devices play a crucial role in furthering healthcare and also for meeting the needs of prevention and provision of clinical care through investigation, diagnosis, treatment, management, follow up and rehabilitation. An unsafe medical product or a product of dubious quality could be a major health

---

[6.] Bandhua Mukti Morcha vs. Union of India (AIR 1984 SC 802).

hazard, given the potency of modern medicines.[7] The world has witnessed many disasters whose origins could be traced to quality compromises.

Ensuring affordability of medical products is another important aspect that has to be addressed by the national governments. It encompasses creation of an eco-system that is conducive for the industry to acquire the required competence and scale and also the establishment of robust quality control and assurance mechanisms. The right to health will not mean much to a person who needs a quality medical product, but is instead provided a substandard quality product that could aggravate the disease burden or even snatch away the life.

The widespread and all-encompassing nature of pandemics, such as COVID-19, also underpins the need for global cooperation and a multilateral strategy. In a globalized world, the inability of any state to efficiently respond to such emergencies would be a serious threat to the population of all other countries. 'No one is safe till everyone is safe' is the motto with which pandemics or any other major global health emergencies or other serious health concerns need to be approached and managed to avoid unbearable costs in terms of human health and lives. Pandemics and other health emergencies do not respect national boundaries and will continue to surface from time to time given, *inter alia*, the fact that humans are wired to experiment with nature, and such experimentation has its own perils, including devastating ones. These might be unintentional or sometimes intentional actions such as letting the biological organisms used in experiments in laboratories out into the environment.

Every crisis is also an opportunity to sit back and ponder over what could have been done better or should be done now to make things better. The breakout of the COVID-19 pandemic succinctly highlights this point. It is not that the human race is witnessing a pandemic for the first time and though one would have wished to see no more pandemics, COVID-19 is certainly not the last one. We need to be prepared for more such crises

---

[7.] The use of heparin API for making formulations detailed in Chapter 9 and thalidomide in Chapter 7 may be referred to.

in the future. There is no universal best way to manage all pandemics, epidemics or other major health crisis. The availability of the state-of-the-art infrastructure and quality resources, both human and material, can, however, help reduce the adverse impacts, including mortality in the aftermath of any such crisis. As part of the social contract between the State and the citizen, it is an obligation of the modern nation states to cater for all these and more.

The COVID-19 crisis has, amongst others, drawn the global attention to the need for continued investment in many vital components of healthcare delivery and increased research & development in healthcare science and technology-related areas globally for expanding the frontiers of human knowledge and developing sustainable and efficient solutions for handling any future pandemics, epidemics or other major health-related emergencies. The endeavor will need to be intensified, and adequately funded through collaboration between different stakeholders.

The advancements in the field of science and technology have led to a paradigm shift in the way new treatments, therapies, vaccines, drugs or even medical devices are developed in a highly compressed time-frame. The vaccine for flu pandemic that started in 1918 could be made available to the general population only in 1945. It took nearly twenty years for developing a vaccine for polio virus after the research for it began in 1935. As contrasted with this, the development of vaccines for COVID-19 has been possible in around two months from the date the details of its genetic code became available.

The large pool of research that had gone into developing other vaccines earlier has been used effectively for finding solutions for COVID-19. In fact, most solutions for handling COVID-19 emerged from past investments in healthcare- related areas. But for such past investments, the situation would have been much more catastrophic. This brings home the importance of continuing and stepping up research & development activities, attaining technological maturity and clear identification of processes, techniques and tools for effectively preventing and, if prevention is not feasible, for tackling similar future challenges to human health.

The crisis also highlights the need for developing the capacity to respond quickly to such health emergencies, including by stepping up the availability of quality medicines, vaccines or medical devices. Infrastructure facilities, such as hospital beds and intensive care units and competent and qualified healthcare professionals both in the urban settings and rural and remote areas, are vital components for effective delivery of healthcare services in such emergencies. There is a need for building a strong cadre of competent human resources for undertaking research, handling clinical aspects and a large set of well-informed and trained frontline health workers to handle diverse aspects, such as initial screening of cases for referrals, disseminating information about non-pharmacological interventions and mobilizing the community to participate in the process of preventing the spread of diseases. The criticality of quality medical products and the ability to use them efficiently can be gauged from the fact that their absence can hamper the outcomes and render the best infrastructural facilities and human resources futile.

Medical products are no longer what they used to be in the olden times. Pharmaceuticals have traveled a long distance from those days when medicines were largely based on intuition and observation. The trial-and-error methods were used to ascertain which plant or animal or mineral contained medicinal qualities. This was followed by an era in which isolation and purification of compounds and chemical synthesis formed the basis of drug discovery and development. Convergence of research in the fields of chemistry and physiology and application of computer-aided design further improved the accuracy and precision of medicines. Small molecular therapeutics, biologicals and biosimilars are the latest tools in the armory of humans to fight the dreaded diseases. The potency of new medical products makes it imperative to ensure that their quality is not compromised.

Before moving on to the substantive chapters, it is considered necessary to introduce the Indian medical products industry briefly. The Indian pharmaceutical industry has been a major success story and the growth has been unstoppable. In 1990 the industry was worth US $1 billion and by 2025, it is estimated to be in the vicinity of US $ 100 billion. Similarly, the

Indian medical devices sector has been growing very fast and is also expected to scale new heights in the near future. The growth of the pharmaceutical industry has helped generate massive employment opportunities in India. Backed by solid fundamentals, the Indian medical products industry is progressively growing in confidence. The responsibility of the Indian pharmaceutical industry has also increased multifold with its growth and the continuous accretion to knowledge and upward revision of the quality requirements by importing countries has also put pressure on the Indian industry.

While details of the scope of the Indian pharmaceutical sector and its reach have been captured in Chapter 1, the growth of the pharmaceuticals industry in post-independent India can be bracketed in four broad stages. The first stage was up to 1970. It was marked by domination of the Indian market by foreign drug manufacturers whose formulations were imported and marketed in the country.

In the second phase (between 1970 and 1990), a large number of domestic manufacturers entered the pharmaceutical manufacturing field. The growth of the sector was spurred by the provisions of the Indian Patents Act, 1970. Growth during this period was also haphazard in view of the non-existence of stringent regulatory structures.

The third phase (1990–2010) witnessed a move towards exports. With the adoption of product patents in 2005, India became a major generic drug manufacturer.

After 2010, India has also entered the biosimilars and biologics arena in a big way. India is currently one of the largest players in the field of biosimilars and biologics. Patented products, consumer healthcare, biologics and biosimilars, vaccines and public health are the areas that appear to be throwing up many new opportunities.

The inspections by regulators of countries importing drugs from India have also progressively helped the Indian industry to increase adherence with the global best practices. However, it has also given rise to two different levels of quality of medical products in the Indian pharmaceutical industry: one catering to the requirement of countries with stringent regulatory requirements and the other for domestic and less-regulated markets. The

Indian pharmaceuticals industry has attracted severe criticism at the hands of drug regulators of importing countries, whistleblowers and the journalist, etc. Chapter 1 captures the criticism of the Indian pharmaceutical industry in detail. Many critics have dubbed the Indian pharmaceutical industry as being responsible for impoverishing the already poor and pushing them to destitution.

The two incongruous descriptions, namely the disparagement of the Indian pharmaceutical industry and the admiration for it, are not unusual. Humans have a tendency to believe their limited, subjective experiences as the absolute and the only truth; they tend to ignore or even dismiss the experiences of others, which might be equally true. An ancient Indian parable is pertinent in this context. In it, a group of blind men who had never come across an elephant earlier, learn and conceptualize what the elephant looked like by touching it. Each man touched or felt only one part of the elephant's body and, coincidentally, that happened to be a part different from what others in the group had touched. Each one of them described the elephant based on their narrow experience. The elephant's description by each one in the group differed.

The present work, in the above background, assesses a number of aspects relating to the Indian pharmaceutical and medical devices industries; their weaknesses, strengths and potential. In doing so, it takes different perspectives into consideration before coming to a conclusion. It also makes recommendations for improving the contribution of the two sectors and prognosticates that augmentation of the quality of medical products could catapult India to be the ultimate destination for global healthcare delivery. It provides an in-depth analysis of how far the Indian industry could contribute to the furtherance of the right to health or constraining its enjoyment. The book has been divided into 11 chapters, and each one of them deals with an identified set of issues. The recommendations to overcome the identified shortcomings have been summed up in an Appendix.

CHAPTER 1

PHARMACEUTICAL INDUSTRY – A VILLAIN OR A SAINT

PHARMACEUTICAL INDUSTRY AND HEALTHCARE DELIVERY

As highlighted in the introduction, accessibility to and affordability of essential medicines and medical devices are crucial for the enjoyment of the right to life, and their non-availability will tantamount to denial of a fundamental human right and also the abdication of the obligation of the State. Medicines, along with other components of healthcare delivery, are important for addressing health-related concerns and improving the quality of human lives. They form an indispensable component for the prevention, diagnosis and treatment of diseases and alleviating disability. Universal health coverage can only be possible with easy access to essential quality medicines and health products, and their affordability.

Combating a myriad of new diseases afflicting human beings requires development of new cures and therapies. For a considerable length of time, the search for new drugs was dependent partly on science and partly on chance. The development of new technologies has led to a paradigm shift in drug discovery and development from a random process to a more precise science. The intersection of physiology, chemistry and information technology tools, including the artificial intelligence and machine learning, and other scientific developments, have made it possible to evolve new therapies that help in developing new medicines for alleviating the pain and misery associated with diseases.

The process of drug discovery and development is full of challenges. On a rough estimate, from out of 8000/10,000 new compounds, only one compound gets approved for marketing and use on human beings. The entire process entails a lot of expenditure and a major chunk of it is borne by the pharmaceutical companies. The quantum of resources committed by pharmaceutical industries to innovation as a percentage of sales is the highest amongst all industries. No other industry commits that kind of resources to innovation.[1] But for the existence of pharmaceutical industry and its role in making medical products available, the very human existence could have been threatened.

It needs to be recognized that business cannot be all philanthropy and for philanthropy also, the funds have to flow in from somewhere. The pharmaceutical industry, much like any other industry, is therefore justified in ensuring a reasonable rate of return on investment so that it can reinvest in further growth. Without reasonable return, no investment and growth can take place. In any case, *sans* pharmaceutical industry, the human and animal life would have been much more miserable. The contribution of the pharmaceutical and medical devices industry can be gauged from the fact that medical products help in sustaining life in many cases where in the absence of these products, death would have been a certainty. It needs to be recognized that the pharmaceutical industry represents the industrial sector as a whole, which in turn represents the society at large. For every good businessperson, there will always be a few of them who might not be outright honest, and that applies to all sections of the society.

CRITICISM OF THE PHARMACEUTICAL INDUSTRY

The honor of being the most criticized industry for reasons that might be justified only partially and can very well be fictitious or imaginary in some instances rightfully belongs to the pharmaceutical industry. The criticism is, however, not confined to the pharmaceutical industry in any one country or only the large pharmaceutical manufacturers; it covers the wide spectrum of institutions, industry and even individuals, ranging from regulators and clinicians to those engaged in research & development and

---

[1.] For more details refer to Chapter 8.

manufacture of branded and generic drugs. The grounds on which the pharmaceutical industry has been criticized are multifarious.

Based on the existing literature, including books and articles in print media on the subject and internet sources, this chapter presents a brief glimpse of such criticism. This, however, is not an exhaustive compilation of the criticism, and the sample has intentionally been confined to the minimum sources so that the reader is not bogged down with far too many details and at the same time, is able to savor its flavor. To the extent necessary and with a view to objectively assess the ground reality, some of the details available with the MoHFW, Government of India have been used to corroborate or contradict the points of criticism.

GLOBAL PHARMACEUTICAL INDUSTRY

The global pharmaceutical industry has been criticized by a cross section of society, including clinicians, researchers, journalists, patient safety networks, etc., for a variety of reasons. Transparency International has in one of its comprehensive assessments titled 'CORRUPTION IN THE PHARMACEUTICAL SECTOR, DIAGNOSING THE CHALLENGES', brought out in 2016, highlighted that there is a scope for corruption at each stage of the journey of pharmaceuticals through the value chain *viz.* the research & development, manufacturing, registration, distribution, procurement and marketing.[2] It has also highlighted some major instances relating to non-transparent and fraudulent practices adopted by many pharmaceutical companies. Details of some of these have been included in the latter part of the chapter.

Dr. Marcia Angell, the former editor of the *New England Journal of Medicine* for two decades, has, in a severe indictment, sought to expose the shocking degeneration in the pharmaceutical industry and argued for essential, long-overdue change in the pharmaceutical practices.[3] The

---

[2] Full text of the report is available at: https://www.transparency.org.uk/sites/default/files/pdf/publications/29-06-2016-Corruption_In_The_Pharmaceutical_Sector_Web-2.pdf

[3] Angel, Marcia: *The Truth About the Drug Companies: How They Deceive Us and What to Do About It.*

author states that pharmaceutical companies have become vast marketing machines that have unprecedented control over their own fortunes and wield undue influence over medical research, education and clinical practices. The often-cited claim that high drug prices fund research & development (R&D), thus leading to discovery of new drugs is, according to Dr. Angell, a big sham and such high prices are actually used for marketing products of dubious benefit.

Drug companies, according to Dr. Angell, rely on publicly funded institutions for basic research; rig clinical trials to make their products look better than what they are; and use legions of lawyers to stretch out government-granted exclusive marketing rights for years. Dr. Angell, keeping this in view, proposes comprehensive reforms, including making clinical research ethical, and delinking drug companies and medical education.

Ben Goldacre has highlighted that the presumption that medicine is based on evidence, fair testing and robust clinical trials, is a big farce.[4] The author argues that, in reality, those tests and trials are often profoundly flawed and critical information is never made available. It argues that much of the research is hidden from doctors who write prescriptions; doctors' education is funded by the pharmaceutical industry; and regulators approve useless drugs, with data on side effects casually withheld from doctors and patients.

In an article titled *Transforming the critique of Big Pharma*, Anne Pollock has highlighted that the intersecting fields of scholarship had accounted for pharmaceutical companies' extraordinary success in promoting and profiting from their wares. The article argues that the pharmaceutical companies do not have complete mastery over the objects they have created. This lack of mastery, it has been argued, has always been present and was merely masked by financial success of pharmaceutical companies.[5] The author concludes that given the potential harm that the

---

[4.] Goldcare, Ben: *Bad Pharma: How Drug Companies Mislead Doctors and Harm Patients*

[5.] Available at https://link.springer.com/article/10.1057/biosoc.2010.44

medical products could cause, the availability of products whose efficacy is not fully established is a serious issue and this could, in many cases, result in more harm than benefit.

Steven Brill has, in his book,[6] commented on the role the pharmaceutical industry plays in gutting price controls. The trade group Pharmaceutical Research and Manufacturers of America (PhRMA), it has been pointed out, spends a lot of money on lobbying. It states that a multibillion-dollar deal with PhRMA, major unions and other liberal groups as part of the Obamacare, manifest the power of PhRMA in influencing public policy.

In addition to the criticism in different books and articles, malpractices of many global pharmaceutical manufacturing units have been documented. The available evidence suggests that the use of unfair means by pharmaceutical companies for promotion of drugs is something not confined to India and the innovator companies outside India are equally complicit. A few sample cases often cited to buttress this include GlaxoSmithKline (GSK) pleading guilty to unlawful promotion of a drug for depression amongst children below 18 years of age even when it knew that it causes suicidal tendencies,[7] and the case of Johnson & Johnson pleading guilty for the use of Risperdal for elderly dementia patients and children with mental disabilities[8]. Both paid hefty penalties when they were found wanting.

Instances such as influencing medical research, and prescribing behavior of physicians, misrepresentation of risks and benefits of drugs, controlling the way research is published, guest-authoring, payments to physicians in cash or kind, sponsoring travels or hotel stay of doctors or workshops and data manipulation are reported to be common global

---

[6.] AMERICA'S BITTER PILL, Money, Politics, Backroom Deals, and the Fight to Fix Our Broken Healthcare System

[7.] The case relates to the clinical trial of Paxil. Details are available at: https://www.justice.gov/opa/pr/glaxosmithkline-plead-guilty-and-pay-3-billion-resolve-fraudallegations-and-failure-report.

[8.] The case related to the promotion of Risperdal for elderly dementia patients and children with mental disabilities by J&J and its subsidiary without USFDA approval. Details available at: https://www.justice.gov/opa/pr/johnson-johnson-pay-more-22-billion-resolve-criminal-and-civilinvestigations.

practices in the pharmaceutical industry. There is a lot that has been written about the negative facets of pharmaceutical and medical devices industry. Some literature – especially with regard to the use of pre-used medical devices – also highlights the lack of ethics and also the covetousness of businesspersons for marketing such products, notwithstanding the possible harm from their reuse. It has been highlighted that in many cases such devices have not been calibrated properly and that could result in wrong diagnosis and inappropriate treatment.

The global pharmaceutical industry has been painted by many as substantially concerned only with minting profits even if it be at the cost of public health. It is considered that even the most balanced approach to assessing the contribution of the global pharmaceutical industry has not been very charitable and in the process, the contribution of the sector for improving health outcomes has largely been ignored. At the same time, it is a fact that the positive contribution of the sector has not been projected to the same extent as that does not attract as much attention as projecting the negative aspects would. Humans are wired to pay more attention to the negative and the unusual. That is why the young journalists were told that the dog biting the man is not as great a news as the man biting the dog would be.

VIBRANT INDIAN PHARMACEUTICAL INDUSTRY

The Indian pharmaceutical industry is one of the most vibrant sectors of Indian economy with a global presence. It is the third largest producer of pharmaceuticals in terms of volume and the 10th largest in terms of value[9] in the world. Indian pharmaceuticals industry contributes 3.5% of total drugs and medicines exported globally. Currently, around 11,000 companies are engaged in manufacturing pharmaceuticals in India.

Over 80% of antiretroviral drugs used globally to combat Acquired Immune Deficiency Syndrome (AIDS) are supplied by the Indian

---

[9.] The rank in terms of value varies in different sources and is stated to be between 10 and 13.

pharmaceutical industry. Similarly, WHO pre-qualified vaccines manufactured in India are exported to nearly 160 countries. The export destinations for pharmaceutical products include countries ranging from the poorest to the most advanced countries of the world.

Apart from generic drug formulations, pharmaceutical exports from India include bulk drugs, intermediates, biologicals, Ayurvedic, herbal products and surgicals. Indian drugs save millions of human lives across continents and improve the quality of many more by enhancing affordability and access to medicines. There could be no doubt that by making generic versions of the costly drugs available at a fraction of the cost of medicines from the innovator companies, the Indian pharmaceutical industry has positively impacted the health economics and health outcomes across the globe.

Given the economic disparities, widespread poverty and deprivation in many countries, a large segment of the global population cannot afford innovator drugs. Besides, the governments of most countries providing free or concessional healthcare will not be able to meet the huge expenditure that the costly innovator drugs entail. In this backdrop, less costly but equally safe and efficacious generic medicines go a long way in mitigating the sufferings of the not-so-privileged sections of the society, especially the poorest, which need these medicines the most.

It would not be out of context to say that the only other Indian sector with a global imprint is the Information Technology and related services. Both these sectors have demonstrated how private enterprise can help in generating employment, reducing costs, increasing production and productivity as also improving profits while meeting global requirements. The scale of the Indian IT/ITES sector is, however, nowhere closer to the top in the world. The Indian pharmaceutical sector, on the other hand, has positioned itself, at least in the case of generic medicines, almost at the top.

The contribution of the Indian pharmaceutical sector has been acknowledged by the UN Secretary General in the context of usefulness of the production facilities for vaccines and medicines in India, particularly to meet the COVID-19 pandemic. It must, however, not be ignored that in both these sectors, the focus has so far been confined largely to what could be termed as the easier part. The hardcore activities, including R&D at the cutting edge of technology, have not been taken up in India to a large extent.

CRITICISM OF THE INDIAN PHARMACEUTICAL INDUSTRY

Since India is a dominant player in the global generic pharmaceutical landscape, it has come up for a much closer scrutiny and pungent criticism for a variety of reasons. Critics have commented adversely on the role of the Indian pharmaceutical industry and magnified a plethora of concerns, especially about the quality of Indian drugs. The severest indictment of the Indian pharmaceutical industry comes from the USFDA, which undertakes the largest number of inspections of the Indian pharmaceutical manufacturing plants as the USA happens to be the single largest importer of generic medicines from India.

It is not that those adverse observations about the Indian pharmaceutical industry are confined only to the USFDA; regulators of other importing countries who conducted inspections of the pharmaceutical manufacturing units in India also found the Indian industry practices wanting in many respects. Concerns about the quality of Indian drugs falling short of meeting the prescribed parameters have, as such, been flagged by a number of countries. However, with some degree of subjectivity, the observations of the USFDA available on its website are, by far, the best guide of what is wrong with the Indian pharmaceutical sector. Such criticism, however, needs to be seen in a broader context as explained in a subsequent section.

If one has to go beyond the reports of drug regulators, a detailed account of the compromises made by generic manufactures, contract research organizations, etc., in furtherance of the rampant corporate greed, and lax standards and inadequate regulatory oversight have been captured by Katherine Eban in a book reported to be the result of investigative journalism.[10] In the harshest possible indignation, the book highlights that

---

[10.] Eban, Katherene: *BOTTLE OF LIES, The Inside Story of the Generic Drug Boom*

rather than acting as global equalizers by making the same cure available to the wealthy and the impoverished, the generic drugs have turned out to be the ultimate subversion and exploitation, making the worst medicines for the poorest patients, with life and death consequences for all.[11]

The author has also pointed out that most manufacturers have different facilities for highly regulated markets and lesser or non-regulated markets, including for domestic consumption in India. It brings out that a large number of complaints have continued to be received against the generic versions of medicines in the USA. It narrates how the patients who had been administered generic versions of medicines suffered while the same patient when given the branded medicine showed improvement. The book recounts the horrific details of problems with the Indian pharmaceutical manufacturing units, some deliberate and others a consequence of the alleged absence of work culture or lack of capacity.

Based largely on the work of Dinesh Thakur (the whistleblower in the case of Ranbaxy), the book also highlights the problems of fabricated documentation at manufacturing sites of many pharmaceutical manufacturers in India, including with respect to tests for dissolution, stability and copying of chromatograms of reference drugs and recording the results as that of the drugs manufactured in-house by the company. It also mentions instances of extraneous material being found in the bulk drugs that was sought to be hidden. It goes on to highlight that the tablets made from that substandard bulk drug were exported to poor countries and the workers were found to be following unhygienic/unsafe practices.

The book narrates that even after being given a chance to rectify mistakes, the corrective actions were not taken in many cases, and data integrity was sorely lacking. The book also uses the reports of the USFDA inspectors selectively to buttress the conclusions drawn by the author. In the process, the author has also found fault with the working of the USFDA.

In the light of such strong indignation, it is necessary to have a clearer picture of the factual position at the ground level. Some of the concerns

---

[11] Ibid page 351(Based on the report of USFDA inspector)

expressed by foreign regulators and others are for real and reflect lack of competence, capacity and even collusion between multiple regulators in the country and the industry it regulates. It is also a fact of life that a number of facilities manufacturing medicines for marketing in India and other non-regulated markets are in poor shape with all kinds of violations of Good Manufacturing Practices (GMP). The concerns regarding dissolution/stability, assay and lack of evidence for pharmacological equivalence are for real.

It is also a fact that many of the concerns have been magnified multifold deliberately to keep the pressure on the Indian pharmaceutical industry for extracting the best value for money. It also needs to be acknowledged that there are a very large number of manufacturers whose manufacturing units have been inspected repeatedly, and their processes and products meet the best global practices. It requires no genius to discern that the drugs would not have been continued to be imported by so many developed countries if they did not meet the prescribed standards and quality parameters. To presume that the stringent regulators of many importing countries did not do their homework properly would be preposterous. This issue has been examined in more details in a subsequent section.

TRADERS AS MANUFACTURERS

Most large private pharmaceutical companies were set up in India to cope with the fast growing domestic and international demand for pharmaceutical products, especially the generic medicines. Blinded by the lure of the international market and profits, some pharmaceutical manufacturers in India adopted shortcuts resulting in quality compromises. The fact that regulators in India were not stringently enforcing norms/GxPs and a number of manufacturers could violate them with impunity encouraged other manufacturers to follow suit.

A unique characteristic of the Indian pharmaceutical industry is that a number of entities who were earlier engaged in trading pharmaceutical products also entered the manufacturing arena keeping in view the fact that they could take up manufacturing without much difficulty as adhering to the requirements, such as stability of the product during its shelf life,[12] therapeutic equivalence[13]/ bioequivalence[14]/bioavailability, etc.[15] were not insisted upon by health authorities and regulators.

An association of drug manufacturers representing a large number of smaller manufacturers has been advancing the narrative that pharmaceutical equivalence is sufficient for ensuring the quality of medicines and insistence on bioequivalence/therapeutic equivalence and other requirements, such as stability during shelf life, were being imposed to oust the smaller units from the manufacturing process. Though in terms of value and volume, their contribution is not more than 10% of the total production of pharmaceuticals in India and 95% of their produce is used for meeting domestic requirements, the associations sometimes use their numerical strength and political clout for perpetuation of the 'Not of Standard Quality' (NSQ) products in the market. It is also a fact that bioequivalence may not be required in all cases; however, it must be adhered to where it is necessary.[16]

The system of lowest bidder (L-I), i.e., the product with lowest price followed in government procurements helps many such units to sustain their profitability. The degeneration in the system can be gauged from the fact that many pharmaceutical units operate only for part of the year and manufacture products exclusively for meeting the requirements of the government. The findings of the largest ever drug survey ever conducted and discussed in detail in a later chapter demonstrate prevalence of very

---

[12.] Shelf life is the period of time during which a pharmaceutical product, if stored as indicated on the label, is expected to comply with the specification as determined by stability studies on a number of batches of the product. The shelf life is used to establish the expiry date of each batch.

[13.] Therapeutic equivalence implies that the drug meets the criteria of both the pharmaceutical equivalence as well as bioequivalence.

[14.] Bioequivalence means the absence of a statistically significant difference in the rate and extent of absorption of an active ingredient from a pharmaceutical formulation in comparison to the reference formulation having the same active ingredient when administered in the same molar dose under similar conditions.

[15.] Bioavailability is the extent and rate at which the active drug enters systemic circulation. Through this process, it reaches the site of action.

[16.] More details in this regard are available in Chapter 4.

high NSQ drugs in government supplies as compared with the samples picked from the market.

It must, however, be admitted that many private sector manufacturers have acted smartly and took steps for integrating quality in the manufacturing processes progressively as they acquired new knowledge as a result of frequent inspections by many international regulators on aspects that were earlier ignored. The improvement in the quality of pharmaceutical products and processes followed in manufacturing of drugs in India is a major contribution of the repeated inspections carried out by foreign regulators. Such inspections also continued to raise the bar, adding layer after layer of the new qualitative requirements to ensure that drugs were sourced at a low cost from India and those also met the highest quality parameters. Today, there are a number of manufacturers who have much better compliance with the requirements than even the manufacturers in advanced countries including in the USA. At the same time, there are drug manufacturers in India – some licensed and others unlicensed – who do not care about quality of their products.

GENERIC MEDICINES AND QUALITY COMPROMISES

Another peculiar feature of the Indian governance model is that while pursuing populist policies, many demagogues who do not understand science, influence both public opinion and public policy. The twisted and deliberate misuse of the term 'generic' in India is one example of such demagoguery. The term 'generic' in the context of medicines essentially refers to the medicines other than the innovator drugs, which are therapeutically as well as pharmaceutically equivalent to the innovator drug. A large number of manufacturers in India manufacture medicines that have only pharmaceutical equivalence and their bioequivalence or therapeutic equivalence has not been established. Many of these have been approved by regulators in the state concerned without proper evaluation of their safety and efficacy. Further, in many cases, even the stability of the drugs over the shelf life has not been established.

The insistence of the government on only generic name of the medicine being put in the label of the drug obfuscates the difference between a drug that is therapeutically and pharmaceutically equivalent to the innovator drug and the one that is only pharmaceutically equivalent. Statements made by different ministers about only generic medicines being prescribed, etc., add to the confusion as generic medicines are confused with cheaper versions that have not gone through required processes such as stability or bioequivalence studies.[17] Such irresponsible statements encourage use of medicines whose quality, safety and efficacy have not been established. The medicines that are not therapeutically equivalent and stable over their shelf life are nothing more than dangerous concoctions that could do more harm than good to the humans and animals.[18]

MANUAL PROCESSES

The issue of data integrity has haunted the Indian pharmaceutical industry as this aspect has specifically been targeted by drug inspectors from importing countries. Many Indian pharmaceutical manufacturers still rely on paper-based processes that are imprecise, slow and cumbersome. The industry populates its batch records manually. In a few cases, a hybrid system with some digitalization has been adopted for inputting data. This, however, is no improvement over the paper-based approach and creates conditions that will allow the defects to slip in.

Manually inputting data introduces human error that, *inter alia*, impacts the recall process adversely and opens up the scope for suspicion, even in cases where the processes are duly followed. It is therefore necessary to move on to complete automation for generation and recording of data. The compromises made by the Indian industry in terms of non-adoption of proper processes, non-compliance with GxP, data integrity and other frauds tumbling out during the inspections by drug regulators of importing countries do no good

---

[17.] For details see Chapter 6.
[18.] This aspect has been covered in more detail in Chapter 6.

to the reputation of the so-called pharmacy of the world. In fact, the problem of the Indian pharmaceutical industry is that it has grown in a haphazard manner and in the absence of well-structured and functional regulatory machinery, qualitative aspects have largely been ignored.[19]

USFDA INSPECTIONS AND OBJECTIVITY

Inspections rarely highlight strengths as they are essentially structured as fault-finding exercises. At the same time, no inspection, howsoever thorough it might be, can detect all deficiencies. Therefore, all inspections highlight only the shortcomings and that is what the USFDA inspections also do. Reports of an inspection cannot be treated as the gospel truth amongst others, for the reason that, firstly, the knowledge of inspectors is limited and they cannot be expected to know everything; and secondly, the inspectors have their angularities that are ingrained in their persona by their upbringing, knowledge and training provided to them and their belief system. It would be absurd to believe that all inspections are always fair and objective. Nevertheless, the mere fact that an inspection has been planned acts as a catalyst for self-introspection and could result in removal of deficiencies by the manufacturer *suo motto*.

Based on the perusal of some inspection reports and keeping in view the cultural and other differences, it would not be out of place to mention that the USFDA inspectors have their own biases that influence the methods adopted by them for carrying out inspections. The Indian industry has continued to raise the issue of such inspections not being always fair, objective and transparent with the MoHFW. Industry claims that many USFDA inspections – unconventional as they were –started with the presumption that the Indian manufacturers were deceiving. It is argued that in most cases they failed to contextualize the differences between practices in India and the USA. It should also not be forgotten that USFDA officials were identifying sources of drugs conforming to the

---

[19.] Chapters 2 and 3 may be seen for more details.

standards of the USA at Indian prices and if they pointed out deficiencies, it was part of their job to do so in furtherance of their national interests, which was to get the best medicines at the least possible prices.

Inter alia, the job of a regulator entails assessing the pros and cons of inspection findings in the light of scientific and other evidence and undertaking benefit *vs.* harm analysis of the proposed courses of action, before taking a final decision. The fact that the USFDA did not approve many findings of its own inspectors, confirms that inspection reports are just one set of inputs that regulators take into account while assessing a facility or a product. Without evidence to the contrary, it would be unreasonable to expect that the USFDA would compromise on issues that impact the health of US citizens. It has, however, been argued that some USFDA inspectors have been treating Indian drug manufacturers unfairly and using all kinds of tactics to target junior employees who do not understand English.

As is usual, the shortcomings get magnified manifold for various reasons like global competition for the generic market, the greed of big pharma in the face of declining market for branded drugs due to the availability of low-cost generic versions and electronic media's obsession with the TRP. Excessive reliance only on what drug inspectors reported is not sufficient to conclude that all generics are bad. It also needs to be noted that the USFDA inspections result in adverse findings in case of even the best administered manufacturer in the USA also and such adverse findings and the warning letters are not unique to the Indian manufacturers.

As far as the account of Dinesh Thakur is concerned, it is sufficient to say that he has done an excellent service both to the Indian pharmaceutical industry and the humanity at large by bringing the serious concerns to limelight and it is now for the Indian authorities to take remedial steps. Thakur still continues to pursue various issues that impinge upon quality of medical devices vigorously. Many in the Indian pharmaceutical industry argue that the account of Dinesh Thakur was highly exaggerated and was influenced by the lure of big money. It would be unfair to discount the persistent efforts made by Dinesh Thakur towards highlighting the major shortcomings of the Indian pharmaceutical sector. Even presuming that considerations of big money as a whistle blower from the USFDA could have played a role in his actions and he did not do it exclusively as a public-spirited person, his contribution had the positive impact of more attention being paid to the quality of pharmaceutical products across the Indian manufacturing plants. It also needs to be understood that the case of Ranbaxy cannot be the reference point for all times to come. A lot of water has flown down the Ganges since then and not taking many such positive changes into account, would be unfair to the Indian industry.

DUAL STANDARDS FOR EXPORT AND DOMESTIC MARKETS

The inspections by drug regulatory authorities in India corroborate that different standards of manufacturing were prevalent in the facilities that were in close vicinity of each other and owned by the same manufacturers. The ones for the regulated markets, such as the USA and Western Europe, were neat, clean, tidy and had state-of-the-art machines with no human intervention from the stage of feeding the raw material into the machines to the packing of the final product. The other ones that catered for domestic and lesser-regulated markets included some steps where the material was also being handled manually. The risk-based inspections undertaken by the Central Drug Standard Control Organization (CDSCO) also corroborate this fact.[20] This brings out the need for better regulation even for domestic markets, which as Chapter 2 brings out, is presently dysfunctional.

CORRUPTION AND DRUG REGULATORY SYSTEM

The global pharmaceutical industry is vulnerable to corruption[21] and bribery. It pervades both the public and private sector, and though its

---

[20.] For details, please refer to Chapter 4.
[21.] Transparency International defines corruption as "the abuse of entrusted power for private gain". Available at: https://www.transparency.org.uk/sites/default/files/pdf/publications/29-06-2016-Corruption_In_The_Pharmaceutical_Sector_Web-2.pdf

nature and scale will vary, it is prevalent across countries. Corruption is typically linked to the exercise of discretion in a prejudicial manner by officials. Unbridled discretion throws up ample opportunities for abuse of power and many scheming entities trap the officials by extending money or other favors to them in exchange for help in accomplishing their activities. Just like the corona virus, corruption mutates, evolves and adapts easily to the changing circumstances and is highly contagious. It has the effect of diverting resources as an illegal gain to an individual. It erodes the efficiency and sustainability of a healthcare system by permitting marketing of substandard medical products, leading to consequences such as serious adverse events, increased morbidity and mortality.

As far as the Indian pharmaceuticals industry is concerned, a host of factors help in creation of an environment conducive for breeding corruption. These include the sub-optimal legal framework; the lax regulatory oversight mechanism; inadequate number of regulatory staff and the quality of human and other resources made available to drug regulatory structures; the pressure on the prices of pharmaceutical products; the greed and covetousness of some businessmen and the wide discretion exercised by regulatory officials, especially in enforcement of law.

In India, widespread malpractices have been noticed in various processes ranging from grant of licenses for drug manufacturing, their storage and transportation; clinical trials, bioequivalence studies, etc. Besides the infamous case of Ranbaxy that resulted in the company pleading guilty in the USA, the evidence gathered during the largest-ever drug survey undertaken anywhere in the world, the findings of risk-based inspections and the results of inspection of bulk drug storage facilities in Delhi (covered in detail in a later chapter), corroborate this conclusion. The existence of a large number of drug manufactures operating without a valid license; manufacturing taking place in non-GMP compliant facilities; grant of licenses for fixed dose combinations (FDCs) without the approval of the product by the CDSCO, etc., could not have been possible without being facilitated by drug regulatory structures on account of some kind of a *quid pro quo*.

The fact that a large number of samples picked up from the government healthcare facilities failed more often than the samples picked up from the market sources speaks volumes about the serious problems in governmental procurement processes.

The malpractices adopted by manufacturers for marketing their products include costly gifts in cash and kind, sponsoring foreign trips and conferences and other events to influence the prescribing behavior of practitioners. To curb the malpractices, the Department of Pharmaceuticals has been working on developing and enforcing a uniform code of pharmaceutical marketing practices (UCPMP). However, this has remained a work-in-progress for nearly a decade now.

The connivance at the state level is much higher as major activities concerning drug manufacturing, licensing, registration, distribution, procurement and marketing within the country are handled by the states, and hence, the opportunity for misuse of authority is far greater. A few cases have been recapitulated here to peep into the level of corruption in drug regulatory structures.

A Drug Inspector of the CDSCO posted in Mumbai who had not even completed his probation in the organization, made it a practice to visit manufacturing plants unannounced, especially on Saturdays and Sundays. He would pick up random issues to pressurize manufacturers and threaten them that action will be taken against them for violations. He even filed cases in the courts of law against the manufacturers at his own level, without the matter having been examined by anyone and without any approval of the competent authorities. He signed the affidavits filed in the courts declaring that he had obtained the approval of the competent authority for prosecution and that he was competent to file the case on behalf of the CDSCO.

In July 2016, in a meeting in the MoHFW, an association of pharmaceutical manufacturers mentioned that they were tired of dealing with certain officers of the CDSCO and many state drug regulators who, in industry parlance, were known as ATMs or officers demanding 'All Times Money'. It was indicated that their demand for money was insatiable.

In the month of July 2016 itself, another delegation of pharmaceutical manufacturers from Gujarat, Andhra Pradesh and Telengana complained that the 'Written Confirmations' required for export of drugs to European countries were being delayed by inspecting officials who were demanding money.

The DCG(I) took the decision that all applications for Written Confirmation should be disposed of within a period of two months of the date of receipt of application, and detailed reasons should be recorded in writing where the applications were rejected. He agreed that wherever necessary, officials from other zones will be deputed to complete inspections in a time-bound manner. Zonal heads were informed that they had the option to either clear the cases or reject them and that they will be held personally accountable if decisions were not taken. The regular monitoring worked and the arrears were cleared within a few months. Later on, the process for grant of such confirmations was simplified under the directions of the MoHFW.

Another instance was related to a signed complaint having been received in the MoHFW without the address of the complainant. It alleged that a person would call the industry representatives intimating that their file was stuck up and its clearance can be expedited for a consideration. He made such calls when the files had actually been cleared and had reached him for preparing the order to convey the decision. In response to a telephonic call on his mobile number, the said official proposed a meeting on the same day or the next day at his house in Mayur Vihar, New Delhi. He informed that the consideration would vary keeping in view the nature of clearance required. As necessary details had been obtained, the individual was disengaged with immediate effect even though he tried to pressurize for his continued engagement.

Based on oral complaints received from industry and independent verification of details, a few officials were transferred in 2016 from the key field positions to the CDSCO Headquarters and assigned non-sensitive work where they were not required to interact with industry. The then DGHS tried to intervene in such cases for cancellation of transfers. As reported in the media, on 16.10. 2019, a middle-level official of the CDSCO, who was earlier given non-sensitive work, was arrested by the Central Bureau of Investigation.

Also, as per media reports, a CDSCO Drug Inspector and the Managing Director of a pharmaceutical company had also been arrested on the grounds of alleged conspiracy to 'manage' adverse results of tests and analysis in a government laboratory. Separately, another media report highlighted that the residential and office premises of an official of Himachal Pradesh Drug Control Department were raided by the vigilance department on the allegations of bribe on 23.08.2019. The media also reported that two CDSCO officials were arrested on 18.05.2021 in connection with the alleged demand of bribe from a medical device manufacturer in Ahmedabad.

There is no doubt that some instances of corruption in drug regulations will continue to come to light; however, this does not necessarily mean that corruption is rampant. For every official alleged to be corrupt, there are many who do their job conscientiously and this also applies to officials of drug regulatory structures. In fact, in many cases, they have been putting in their best efforts to restore the semblance of order in the face of all-round anarchy.

MAY NOT BE A SAINT BUT IT IS NOT A VILLAIN EITHER

Notwithstanding the severe condemnation of the pharmaceutical industry, including both the innovators and generic manufacturers at the global level or the Indian industry, it is difficult to agree with all that has been alleged. All said and done, the medicines and medical devices have improved the quality of human life and reduced the adverse impact of debilitating diseases. As of now, there are no proven and efficacious alternatives to the modern medicines and medical devices. While some alternative systems such as Ayurveda, Naturopathy and cellular nutrition have been projected as possible options, these could, at their current stage of development, at best complement medical products.

Cellular nutrition, a unique blend of high-quality bio-available plant-derived nutrients that act at a cellular level and optimize absorption and effectiveness of vitamins and minerals and helps in maintaining proper health,[22] looks more like the intuition in the early stages of development of pharmaceuticals. The logic is that while it may not treat diseases directly, the nutrients given at optimal levels help in achieving the desired health outcomes. It would, however, not be wrong to say that such alternatives cannot be a complete package for managing or curing most diseases.

In the absence of any other viable alternative for prevention, cure and treatment of different ailments, availability of good healthcare system and quality medical products is a prerequisite. The fact remains that medical products will continue to play a critical role in managing concerns relating to human health, and one cannot imagine the world without medicines, at least for the foreseeable future. A number of diseases have been cured, eradicated or eliminated by using medicines. The variety of vaccines that have been developed and marketed to inoculate very large population highlight the positive contribution of the sector towards the well-being of humanity. The efforts made in terms of research, development and drug discovery cannot be ridiculed as mere marketing stratagems.

The pharmaceutical industry is not a static monolith; it comprises heterogeneous manufacturers with different levels of competence, ethics and work culture. Painting the entire industry with the same brush is, therefore, unwarranted and is divorced from the ground reality. At the same time, all claims of pharmaceutical companies cannot be accepted on their face value and some amount of exaggeration on their part cannot be ruled out. There is a grain of truth in many allegations that have been leveled. In case of the Indian pharmaceutical industry, its global reach is now well established; however, the concerns need to be addressed seriously and expeditiously.

On balance of consideration, the pharmaceutical industry – both at the global and the Indian levels –is rendering vital service to the humanity

---

[22.] Ray D. Strand: *What Your Doctor Doesn't Know About Nutritional Medicine.*

and helping in the enjoyment of the right to health and access to essential medicines. It might not be a saint; but it certainly is a hero and not the villain. The distortions on which the criticism of the sector is based are aberrations and not the rule. It is another matter that the level of aberrations is disproportionately high. It should be taken as constructive suggestions for further improvements and helping in evolving sustainable solutions that balance the right to do business and earn legitimate profits, and ensure consumer well-being and wellness.

CHAPTER 2

UNINSPIRING MEDICAL PRODUCTS REGULATION

The quality of medical products plays a crucial role in healthcare delivery. Documented global evidence highlights how disastrous the health consequences of the proliferation of substandard quality drugs could be.[1] No doubt, to ensure the quality of medical products, the internal quality control and quality assurance apparatus in the manufacturing organizations need to be impeccable. The internal quality control and assurance measures within the manufacturing units need to be reinforced by an independent and effective external oversight and monitoring mechanism i.e. a strong and capable National Regularity Authority (NRA) for medical products.

The existence of a robust and efficient NRA in a country enhances public trust in the products and services. The strong NRA also compels the internal quality assurance/control mechanisms and, in fact, the manufacturing unit as a whole to be on the guard and perform their functions more diligently and efficiently. The inefficient drug regulatory structures, on the other hand, result in many more substandard medical products entering the market.

Public health protection is one of the primary mandates of every NRA. The oversight by the NRA at each stage of the product lifecycle impacts healthcare to a significant extent, *inter alia,* through interactions with patients, providers and manufacturers. The medical products regulators are not only responsible for the quality, safety and efficacy of drugs; they also play an important role in healthcare innovation. The drug regulatory structures, therefore, need to be unified, robust, efficient

---

[1.] The case of Heparin API detailed in Chapter 9 may be referred to in this context.

and autonomous; and the officials concerned need to possess the domain knowledge in their respective areas of responsibility such as drugs, medical devices, biologicals, stem cells, regenerative medicine, etc. They should also be conversant with the latest developments in the related scientific fields as also with ethical and legal issues. In addition, the regulator should be able to leverage the expertise available outside the organization in furtherance of its role.

The Indian pharmaceutical industry, manufacturing mainly generic formulations, has witnessed fast-paced expansion during the last three decades. It peaked after 2005. This expansion has helped in generating substantial employment opportunities in India; increased exports that rose even during the global meltdown, including the one induced by the COVID-19 pandemic, and has been a constant source of inward foreign exchange remittances. Globally, the Indian generic drugs have enhanced access to affordable medicines and impacted the health budgets and health outcomes in many countries. It is, in this light that India is often referred to as the pharmacy of the world.

The unimpeachable in-house quality control measures in each manufacturing unit and the robustness of the drug regulatory structures in a country supplying generic medicines across continents is vital for ensuring the safety and welfare of patients globally. The previous chapter captured the details of the criticism of the Indian pharmaceutical sector and a few chapters that follow bring out specific instances of the culpability of Indian drug manufacturers. Chapter 1 recapitulated that the regulators and governments of many countries continue to express concerns about the quality of drugs sourced from India. The large number of inspections undertaken by regulators of countries importing generic medicines from India indicates the lack of global trust in the Indian drug regulatory structures. Similar concerns have also been expressed in other quarters even about the quality of drugs marketed in India.

Overall, in many cases, there are inadequate internal quality assurance/ control systems within the manufacturing units. What is worse is that the drug regulatory authorities in India fail to imbibe confidence for various reasons. As such, there are serious question marks over the robustness and quality of both the internal quality control structures in many manufacturing units as well as the Indian drug regulatory structures. It must however, be clarified at the cost of repetition, that the doubts about the quality of drugs imported by countries with stringent regulations are based on the situation that prevailed over a decade back. With a very large number of inspections having been undertaken by the USFDA and other regulators, the conformance with quality requirements in Indian pharmaceutical manufacturing plants that export drugs to well regulated markets is comparable with or even better than the conformance in most developed countries.

The present chapter assesses the position of the Indian drug regulatory structures and identifies its weaknesses. These, amongst others, are the diffused responsibility with overlapping jurisdictions of the central and state governments; the multiplicity of laws and agencies responsible for nurturing and regulating the sector; lack of coordination; poor human resources management; the inadequacy of resources and inefficient record management. Many of these weaknesses can be traced to the constitutional fault-lines, archaic laws, absence of political will and commitment to reforms, half-hearted efforts at strengthening and reforming the drug regulatory architecture, bureaucratic inefficiency, poor implementation and a host of other factors.

CONSTITUTIONAL FAULT-LINES AND DIFFUSED STRUCTURES

The Constitution of India, like any other constitutions of the world, is not without fault-lines. Some of these also concern the healthcare sector. For example, the subject 'drugs' which includes medical devices, is covered by Entry 19 of List III (Concurrent List) of Schedule 7 of the Indian Constitution. The entry reads as- *'Drugs and Poisons, subject to the provisions of entry 59 of List I with respect to Opium'.* Accordingly, both the central and state governments are competent to take legislative, administrative and other required steps for regulation of drugs in the country. Public health, on the other hand, is included in the state list and the responsibility for that rests exclusively with the states.

The central government plays a pivotal role in the provision of public health through a number of central schemes with massive budgetary outlays. In this regard, it will be educative to also keep the issues related to the COVID-19 management, including procurement of vaccines, in view. In this case, some Chief Ministers raised a pertinent point in May 2021when faced with shortage of vaccines. They sought to draw a parallel and postulated whether in the event of any future war, the states will be left to fend for themselves. Drugs/medicines and public health are closely intertwined and, to that extent, the current placement of the two in the lists under the Seventh Schedule of the Constitution of India is problematic.

The federal polity demands that the remit of the respective governments be honored and as public health falls in the domain of the states, interference by the Centre can legitimately be questioned. There can, however, be no doubt that the solutions for health emergencies cannot be state specific, and that underpins the need for shifting public health to the Concurrent List and drugs to be placed in the Union List. The fact that the international agencies and manufacturers interact only with the federal government lends credence to this argument. The entire flak for not addressing the quality concerns is invariably directed towards the CDSCO, whereas the major responsibility for drug regulation within the country is vested in the states and the CDSCO has limited authority to intervene in such matters.

One of the major concerns regarding the current institutional arrangement relating to medical products regulation in the country is the existence of three dozen-plus central and state regulators having concurrent jurisdiction in the matter. In several instances, the regulators can be found working at cross purposes. It is difficult to visualize any effective drug regulation with such diffused structures and no wonder, the regulation of the quality, safety and efficacy/efficiency of medical products gets sidestepped. The responsibility of all is the responsibility of none. In this situation, the issues that should be accorded high priority get ignored as a consequence of the bystander effect.[2] The confusion and chaos accompanying the diffused responsibility also creates conditions conducive for rent seeking and other malpractices, both on the part of regulators and the regulated.

MULTIPLICITY OF LAWS AND POLICIES

Drug regulation has a large number of facets and a number of laws have been enacted and policies enunciated from time to time for dealing with regulation of medical products. In the absence of harmonization, sometimes, such multiplicity results in contradictory provisions being included in different laws, policies and practices. The major laws that deal with the subject include, 'The Drugs & Cosmetic Act, 1940'; 'The Pharmacy Act, 1948'; 'The Drugs and Magic Remedies (Objectionable Advertisements) Act, 1954'; 'The Narcotic Drugs and Psychotropic Substances Act 1985'; 'The Patent Act'; and 'The Medicinal and Toilet Preparations (Excise Duties) Act, 1956'. The first three legislations are administered by the MoHFW as they primarily concern health-related issues. The major executive orders and policies include the Drugs (Prices Control) Order (DPCO) 1995 under the Essential Commodities Act as amended from time to time to cover specified dosages and strengths as included in the relevant National List of Essential Medicines (NLEM); The National Pharmaceutical Pricing Policy, 2012; and The National Health Policy, 2017. It will be desirable to have a fresh look at all these laws, policies and other executive orders, and harmonize them or may be, reduce their numbers. Keeping in view its focus, most of these Acts, executive orders and policies are not proposed to be covered in detail keeping in view the scope of the present work.

[2.] Bystander effect refers to the phenomenon in which the greater the number of persons present, the lesser the likelihood of action being taken by anyone.

DRUGS& COSMETICS ACT, 1940

The Drugs Act, 1940, as it was titled when enacted on the recommendations of the Drugs Enquiry Committee Report submitted in March 1931, is a pre-independence legislation. It was enacted in pursuance of the long-felt need for regulating the quality, safety and efficacy of drugs in the country in the pre-independence era. This law had been enacted keeping in view the provisions of the Government of India Act, 1935 that vested the provinces with much more authority than what would have been vested in them under the Constitution of India. Hence, the Drugs & Cosmetics Act, 1940 does not appropriately reflect the current constitutional provisions and is an anachronism of a bygone era based on the vestiges of the pre-independence governmental architecture.

In accordance with the archaic Drugs & Cosmetics Act, 1940, the responsibility for drug regulation in India is concurrently exercised by the central and state governments through the Central Drugs Standard Control Organization (CDSCO) and state drug regulators, respectively. As such, three dozen-plus regulators control the quality of medical products in India and each one of them functions independently of the other. The state drug regulators are only subject to the control of the respective state governments and take directions from them. On many occasions, such directions are contrary to the decisions taken by the central regulator and also international practices. It is unthinkable that any country with so many drug regulators acting independently could ensure any uniformity in the regulation of medical products. This is more so as many of them are not even on the same page on many issues, particularly those having political overtones and work at cross purposes in many cases.

As the Drugs Act, 1940 vested the provincial governments with wide powers for drug regulation, rules on the subject were initially framed by different provinces. This gave rise to a plethora of problems in implementation of the law on a pan-India basis. However, before long, it was realized that it would not be possible to have different sets of rules in different states of the country as drugs manufactured in any province would be marketed throughout the country without being subjected to any additional tests or analysis, or cross checking the conformance with the rules framed in the state where such products were to be marketed. The Drugs Act, 1940 was accordingly amended in 1955 and the power to frame rules was exclusively vested in the central government.

Broadly, the Drugs and Cosmetics Act, 1940 vests the central government with the regulatory control over drugs imported in to the country, approval of new drugs, including clinical trials, laying down the standards for drugs and coordination with state regulators for bringing uniformity in drug regulatory practices throughout the country. Through an amendment to the Act, the central government has also been given the overarching power to prohibit, restrict or regulate the import, manufacture, sale and distribution of drugs in public interest, *inter alia*, to take care of public health concerns or to meet health-related emergencies. Most of these functions are discharged through the CDSCO, a subordinate office of the Directorate General of Health Services (DGHS) under the MoHFW.

The state governments exercise substantial control over drug regulation in India. The Drugs & Cosmetics Rules, 1945 delegate a lot of authority to state drug regulators. The state drug regulators have been given the responsibility for licensing manufacturing establishments and sale premises; undertaking inspection of such premises for ensuring compliance with the conditions of license; drawing samples for testing and monitoring the quality of drugs; taking actions such as suspension or cancellation of licenses; surveillance over sale of spurious and adulterated drugs; instituting prosecution when required and monitoring objectionable advertisements for promotion or otherwise of drugs. The regulatory control over manufacture and sale of drugs is exercised through a system of licensing and inspection by state licensing authorities. State drug regulators have, in many cases, also been entrusted with the responsibility of food regulation by state governments. The human and other resources made available to state drug regulatory authorities are nowhere commensurate with the tasks assigned to them either in terms of absolute numbers or from the perspective of quality. This complicates the regulatory responsibilities and often adds to confusion.

Both the CDSCO and state regulators are jointly responsible for grant of licenses in respect of critical drugs such as blood and blood products, I.V. fluids, vaccine and sera. A very loose mechanism for coordination between the central and state authorities has been established in the form of a Drug Consultative Committee (DCC) comprising the central and state regulators. The DCC, however, meets only a few times in a year and that does not necessarily help in better and coordinated regulation.

It has been noticed that some of the state regulators are competent; however, many state regulators do not possess the required skill sets in requisite measure to discharge their responsibility either as members of the DCC or as the state licensing authority. In any case, the deliberations in the DCC are too packed to allow for any meaningful consideration of serious issues. Moreover, many members come unprepared for the meeting. Importantly, the decisions of the DCC have no legal or binding force and, as such, it is no more than a platform for exchange of notes on regulatory issues of current topical interest.

The failure of the central government to amend the Constitution of India or make necessary changes in the laws relating to drug regulation for all these years after the Constitution of India came into force has only compounded the problems. There can be no doubt that the existing arrangement is a sure recipe for disaster as once the responsibility is entrusted to multiple authorities, no single individual or authority can be held accountable. In a situation of diffused responsibility, there is a strong tendency for each individual to assume that someone else will take the responsibility or will do the needful. In reality, no one actually attends to many important activities in such situations.

In the light of the above facts and in the interest of uniformity in drug regulation and for ensuring that safe, qualitative and efficacious medical products are available, the matter relating to centralization of drug regulation in the country has been highlighted many times over in the past. Amongst others, the central regulators, like the rest of the central bureaucracy in

India, are relatively free from local pressures, whether from politicians or industrialists. Such pressures quite often arise from the genuine desire to promote economic activity in the state or generating employment through industrialization. Looked at individually, none of these objectives can *per se* be faulted and they are indeed noble. However, owing to competition between states, they outbid each other and make drug regulation lax. As a result, humanity at large suffers.

The approvals that continued to be granted by ill-equipped state drug regulators for manufacturing fixed dose combinations (FDCs) even decades after the power had been vested exclusively in the central drug regulator demonstrate the culpability of the existing regulatory structures.[3]

Pending resolution of the issues relating to refinement of the Seventh Schedule of the Constitution of India, the central government is competent to take necessary corrective action in such cases under the existing constitutional scheme. Since drugs have specifically been included in the Concurrent List, nothing can stop the central government from enacting a suitable central legislation to address the problematic issues such as multiplicity of regulators. In accordance with Article 254 of the Constitution of India, to the extent of inconsistency between the central and state laws, the central legislation on the subject shall prevail. Needless to say, both the central and state governments in India have been found wanting as far as addressing these issues is concerned.

MULTIPLICITY OF AGENCIES

The multiplicity of agencies involved in medical products regulation is not restricted to centre–state distribution of work and the existence of three dozen-plus regulators. Within each level of government, the responsibility has been assigned to a number of entities. In the central government, the departments involved in the process of regulation of different aspects of medical products include: the Department of Health and Family Welfare;

---

[3] For a detailed analysis of FDCs please refer to Chapter 5.

Department of Health Research; Ministry of Chemicals and Fertilizers, especially the Department of Pharmaceuticals; Ministry of Commerce; Department of Science and Technology; Department of Scientific and Industrial Research; Ministry of Environment, Forests and Climate Change; Department of Biotechnology; Department of Agricultural Research & Education; Ministry of Fisheries, Animal Husbandry and Dairying and a few others too. While the primary responsibility in respect of health-related issues is that of the MoHFW, along with its attached and subordinate offices, other departments are involved in regulating different facets. The Department of Pharmaceuticals is also responsible for promotion of the pharmaceutical and medical devices industry.

The autonomous organizations, attached and subordinate offices involved in the process include the Indian Pharmacopoeia Commission; the National Institute of Biologicals (NIB); Directorate General of Health Services, Indian Council of Medical Research; the Central Drugs Standard Control Organization (CDSCO); the National Pharmaceutical Pricing Authority (NPPA); Laboratories of the Council of Scientific and Industrial Research; Controller General of Patents, etc. Price control mechanism that impacts the quality, accessibility and affordability of drugs is handled by the Nation Pharmaceutical Pricing Authority (NPPA) under the Department of Pharmaceuticals.

The statutory committees that help in the process of drug regulation include the Drugs Consultative Committee (DCC) and Drugs Technical Advisory Board (DTAB). A large number of advisory committees make recommendations on approval of clinical trials of new and investigational drugs. These are: Subject Expert Committees (SEC) comprising experts who advise on clinical trials-related matters, New Drug Advisory Committee (NDAC) headed by Secretary, Department of Health Research, and Investigational New Drugs Committee (INDC) headed by Director General, Indian Council for Medical Research (ICMR). In addition to this, various sub-groups and sub-committees are set up from time to time to deal with specific issues.

The Department of Biotechnology also supports the CDSCO in identifying, formulating, implementing and monitoring various activities related to the application of biotechnology in the field of medical products, including through its Division of Biologicals and the Cellular Biology-Based Therapeutic Drug Evaluation Committee (CBBTDEC). The safety of research projects and activities like small-scale field trials, import, export, clinical trials, etc., involving genetically engineered organisms is monitored and cleared by the review committee on genetic manipulation (RCGM) under the Department of Biotechnology. In many cases, meetings of various committees or expert bodies get organized only after long intervals of time and sometimes, the meetings are not very productive as a lot of time is wasted in discussing issues that are not relevant to the subject. Often the discussions in the committee meetings are monopolized by vocal members.

The CDSCO, as such, is dependent on external inputs for many activities entrusted to it such as evaluation of new drugs, clinical trials, and clearances required from biological and environmental angles. Since this work is not the primary mandate of other organizations rendering external assistance, the task does not get sufficient priority in their scheme of things. Further, in some cases, these committees do not necessarily have the competence to make significant improvements in the regulatory practices. Rationalization on this count should include creation of some internal expertise in the CDSCO. In brief, though some degree of dependence on external agencies cannot be obviated, it is necessary that the CDSCO has the bare minimum human resources to ensure effective coordination in the respective areas.

The regulatory authorities are generally conceived as autonomous institutions having the power to enforce laws or rules on their own without any intervention from other institutions of the State. In other words, they are solely responsible for discharging the responsibility entrusted to them, and only administrative issues are left to be handled by the government. As a subordinate office of the DGHS, the CDSCO has virtually very little autonomy in discharging its responsibility and it is controlled by the

DGHS even with regard to matters where the DGHS does not have the required competence.

STARVING OF INSTITUTIONS

There is yet another important and typical facet of Indian institutional arrangements. The country has been setting up new institutions with very high and laudable objectives. While setting them up, the authorities concerned make very optimistic statements for public consumption. In most cases, some initial funding is also provided to such institutions. However, the required resources in terms of men, money and material are never made available and the annual budgetary allocations take care of only the minimal requirements. The release of such resources is invariably subject to completion of procedural formalities, and the job of ensuring compliance with such formalities lies with officials who will raise any number of objections and queries, but ensure that the resources do not become available to the institutions in time. The common story has been that of a mismatch between creation of assets and their utilization. In most cases, the government has been unable to appoint suitable officials to head many organizations. It needs no detailed elaboration that an organization cannot deliver its best without the required resources and the non-availability of the top management to steer the organization substantially handicaps any such organization. This is a major area of concern and is not restricted to one organization or agency.

As brought out earlier, the primary responsibility for regulating medical products is shared by the CDSCO and state drug regulators. In most cases, these structures – both at the centre and the states – are operating broadly at one-third or one-fourth of the sanctioned manpower, and with poorly equipped laboratories and other infrastructural limitations. The situation in most states is worse than in the Centre. It is, however, not proposed to cover the state-specific issues in detail in the present work as it is premised on the belief that multiple regulatory structures need to give way to a unified central regulator.

A few other organizations that support the drug regulatory structures are equally badly placed and these include the Indian Pharmacopoeia Commission and the National Institute of Biologicals. Given the important functions entrusted to them, it will be necessary to briefly assess their roles, competency and inadequacies.

INDIAN PHARMACOPOEIA COMMISSION

The measurement of quality without specifying standards is not possible and standards are meaningless without the authority to enforce them. This sums up the relationship between the Indian Pharmacopoeia Commission and the national drug regulatory structures in India. Pharmacopoeia creates public standards that are used by regulatory authorities to protect public health by controlling the quality of drugs. It provides a handy tool with which an independent judgment regarding the quality of drugs can be made. Pharmacopoeias need to be continuously revised to factor in developments in science and medical practice.

Set up on January 1, 2009 as an autonomous institution under the MoHFW, Indian Pharmacopoeia Commission (IPC) has been assigned the responsibility to lay down the authoritative standards relating to quality of drugs, including active pharmaceutical ingredients, excipients and dosage forms used by health professionals, patients and consumers with a view to promote the highest standards of drugs within the practical limits of the technologies available for manufacture and analysis. It lays down the standards of drugs used both for human and veterinary purposes. In this process, it regularly publishes Indian Pharmacopoeia and its Addenda; prepares, certifies and distributes IP Reference Substances (IPRS)[4] to stakeholders; publishes National Formulary of India (NFI)[5] for promoting

---

[4.] IPRS are the official standards issued by the Indian Pharmacopoeia Commission (IPC).
[5.] National formulary contains a list of medicines that are approved for prescription throughout the country. It is a guidance document meant for use by healthcare professionals, students, nurses and pharmacists for appropriate selection of medicines. It also indicates which products are interchangeable, and also promotes rational use of generic medicines.

rational use of medicines by healthcare professionals; and undertakes analysis of new drug candidate materials.

It has also been entrusted with the responsibility to administer the Pharmacovigilance Program of India (PvPI) and plays an important role in skill development through hands-on training to regulators, researchers, scientists, analysts, academicians and students in areas related to standard setting for drugs, drug analysis, pharmacovigilance[6] and other related areas. It includes information on the composition, description, selection, prescribing, dispensing and administration of medicines.

Like all other structures, the IPC is also starved of resources. The sanctioned human resources are nowhere close to what is required in a country that supplies medicines to most countries of the world. A number of positions, including that of the Director cum Scientific Secretary of the Commission remained vacant for varying lengths of time.

An ambitious project of the Indian Pharmacopoeia Commission was to set up a state-of-the-art laboratory at its premises in Ghaziabad, UP. The project was sanctioned and necessary funds were made available from 2015 onwards. Unfortunately, while the structure is now in place, the required equipment and manpower have not been provided. The investment, as such, is going down the drain. Similarly, the Pharmacovigilance Program of India is also suffering from lack of adequate human resources and continues to be managed through *ad hoc* arrangements.[7] Overall, the commission is ill equipped to discharge its functions efficiently.

National Institute of Biologicals

Biopharmaceuticals[8] are fast emerging as the medicines of the future. Keeping in view the fact that biologics are a diverse class of molecules, competent professionals are required to analyze and characterize these

---

[6.] Pharmacovigilance is a system comprising activities relating to the detection, assessment, understanding and prevention of adverse effects or any other drug-related problem.

[7.] For details see Chapter 7.

[8.] Biopharmaceuticals are pharmaceuticals manufactured by using biotechnological methods.

products.[9] Set up in 1992, the National Institute of Biologicals (NIB), an autonomous institute under the administrative control of the MoHFW, Government of India, is responsible for promoting and protecting human health by monitoring and ensuring the quality, efficacy and safety of biological products. As the National Control Laboratory in the field of biologicals, including vaccines, diagnostics, blood products, rDNA products, etc., NIB is responsible for developing monographs for these products for inclusion in the Indian Pharmacopoeia, and ensuring uniform standards.

The diverse character of biologicals and non-availability of reference standards is a major challenge for ensuring uniformity in regulating these products. The role of the NIB in promoting and protecting public health by ensuring both access to and affordability of high-quality biologics such as therapeutics, diagnostics and vaccines for the Indian population is critical, especially as the Indian biological sector is on a high-growth trajectory. Given the right impetus, the sector has the potential to turn India into a biopharmaceuticals innovation and manufacturing hub. The availability of human resources with sound technical capabilities for employment in the biopharmaceutical industry and industry–academia linkages is vital for the growth of the biopharmaceutical industry.

Most of the existing educational institutions can provide only limited exposure to design, production, labeling, promotion, manufacturing, testing and regulatory aspects of biologicals. The knowledge about the basic science behind biologics, the potential medicines of the future and the fundamentals of new products is, as such, missing. Inadequate knowledge, lack of hands-on training and absence of competent professional guidance are major handicaps in the development of high-quality human resources required for the sector.

Initially dubbed as a white elephant, NIB has shown a lot of promise in the recent past. However, its potential is not being realized owing to lack

---

9. Biopharmaceuticals are highly complex molecules and are easily affected by changes in the manufacturing process, including temperature fluctuations, making it less active or even inactive.

of vision and inadequate human resources. Some of these concerns have been covered in the next chapter while discussing the corrective action taken or action that had been proposed to be taken but could not fructify.

POOR HUMAN RESOURCES DEVELOPMENT

Competent, confident and trustworthy human resources are the lynchpin for realizing the organizational objectives. It will not be an exaggeration to say that no organization can succeed without the right kind of human resources and more than anything else, the success of any organization hinges largely around the quantity and quality of its manpower. The inadequacy of existing human resources in the drug regulatory structures such as the CDSCO and state drug regulatory authorities, the Indian Pharmacopoeia Commission and the National Institute of Biologicals – in absolute numbers as well as in terms of quality and expertise – is adversely impacting the regulation of medical products. Human resources of the right kind are not always available off the shelf and even if they were, nurturing them will still be required to, *inter alia*, acclimatize them with the organizational culture and ethos, especially in pharmaceutical and medical technology-related areas.

Qualified human resources need to be developed through a meticulous and well-conceived training and developmental strategy as part of the long-term organizational plan, and it needs to be executed efficiently. Investment in structured training and developmental activities helps in nurturing talent and building a culture of pride in the quality of work amongst employees. Training and developmental activities, if planned and executed efficiently, will help in leveraging and multiplying the organization's viability. These contribute both to the growth of the organization and empowerment of employees, and also strengthens trust, imbibes commitment and builds good relationships. The key to successful accomplishment of organizational objective is the right training at the right time.

A good training program empowers employees to take responsibility for the activities of the organization and helps them understand the underlying processes quickly. The systematic nurturing also enhances employees' confidence and taps into their desire for competence, personal development and job satisfaction. While in theory, everyone endorses the need for robust training and developmental activities, the ground reality is different as the capacity building of human resources in most organizations is one of the least understood and most neglected aspects.

Guided by expediency, training and developmental activities, often, get relegated to the bottom of the priority in most organizations. In emergent circumstances, the training and developmental activities would be the first to be dispensed with. Till 2015, there were hardly any structured training and developmental activities for drug regulatory staff and only sporadic training programs were organized. The lack of structured training and developmental activities has also been one of the reasons for the lax and non-uniform regulation of medical products in the country.

POOR LABORATORY INFRASTRUCTURE

The Indian drug regulatory apparatus does not have a robust infrastructure and adequate human resources for ensuring adherence with the strictest quality control/quality assurance processes during various stages of actual manufacturing of medical products. There are hardly any periodic inspections of the manufacturing units and even when inspections are undertaken, they lack depth. In the circumstances, testing and analysis of the finished formulations in the laboratory is the only available alternative to validate the quality of these medical products. Admittedly, testing and analysis of the end products alone cannot assure the quality of medicines. In the absence of quality assurance during manufacturing, the testing and analysis of the end products assumes critical importance for ascertaining the quality of drugs.[10]

Most of the drug testing laboratories of the central or state governments had not been accredited by NABL or certified by ISO till 2014 and nearly all of them had equipment that was either outdated or non-functional.

[10.] For more details on quality-related aspects please refer to Chapter 4.

While the sanctioned posts were much below the requirements, the actual number of officials in positions were even much lower. The central drug testing laboratories at Kolkata, Chennai, Hyderabad and Guwahati do not have full-time Directors even in 2021. The post of Director, Central Drug Laboratory, Kasauli, which tests vaccines and other biologicals, has been filled up by making temporary arrangements. Even the number two and number three positions in most of the drug testing laboratories are vacant.

The position in the states is even worse. Some strengthening of the laboratories had been attempted after 2015; however, the position is still far from satisfactory. In any case, given the reach and scale of the Indian pharmaceutical industry and the consumption of medical products in the country, the number of laboratories and their capacity for tests and analysis is sub-optimal. In a country, that does not have the requisite wherewithal for periodic inspection of manufacturing plants and enforcing process standards, the lack of robust laboratory network for testing and analysis of the end products could have disastrous health consequences in terms of poor quality medical products being sold to the consumers.

POOR RECORD MANAGEMENT

The lack of accountability of structures continues to be one of the serious concerns in the effective regulation of drugs in India, a country that happens to be the largest source of generic medicines sold across the globe. Enforcement of the laws relating to drug regulation in India also suffers on account of poor record management, including its storage and retrieval. Retrieving and using the information that might be available with one of the 37 regulators by any other regulatory authority is completely ruled out in the absence of any centralized system of record keeping. Unfortunate as it is, even within the CDSCO, the retrieval of information maintained manually in multiple files continues to be a horrendous task. The missing files in the CDSCO had been one of the areas that had attracted criticism by the parliamentary committees and also the courts.

Multiplicity of regulators in a country of continental size without any common electronic platform for storage and quick retrieval of information by different regulators poses a lot of problems in handling prosecution or other administrative action or even for the recall of the drugs. The lack of an effective system for coordination between regulators for exchanging information, especially for dealing with any eventuality, only exacerbates the situation. The critics of drug regulatory structures in India cite missing files as a convenient tool to escape responsibility.

It needs to be acknowledged that the process of clearance of proposals, particularly in the case of new drugs or investigational drugs and devices or clinical trials, involves huge data and paperwork. Limited institutional memory and the absence of proper record management make it impossible to retrieve the required information which, in the absence of digitalization, is unfortunately available only in silos. In this scenario, given the pressure of the job and the inadequate staff, if the officials concerned get transferred or leave the job, locating records in the CDSCO becomes nearly impossible. The absence of information makes it difficult to initiate action, especially when the violations happen to be in different states. Poor record management, faulty storage of records and its retrieval cause considerable delays in processing proposals.

To sum up, regulation of medical products in India is currently highly fragmented, multilayered and a diffused process. It would not be wrong to say that the complex web of the existing Indian drug regulatory framework has far too many players to ensure any meaningful regulation. Such diffused regulatory processes permit many defects to seep in through gaps that would not be visible on the face of it. The drug regulatory framework, as it is currently structured, reflects cluttered thought processes. At the least, it manifests non-application of mind and a costly omission to act on an important issue that has continued to give rise to serious concerns, both from domestic and international quarters. To put it mildly, the present medical products regulatory framework in India obfuscates any clarity about who is responsible for regulating the sector. There is no accountability for the consequences of actions or serious omissions or decisions not being made, culminating in adverse events that could jeopardize human life.

It would be worth remembering that the responsibility of all is the responsibility of none, and India can continue to function with such a fractured regulatory structure only at a great disadvantage to billions of people in India and across the globe. Regulation of medical products has to be science-based and that requires suitable augmentation of the resources at the disposal of the CDSCO, including the experts in different domain areas. The consolidation of the entire regulatory edifice into a unified national medical products regulatory authority is also required. It would be unfair to task an expert in pharmaceutical with regulation of engineering products. To complete the story, the next chapter takes stock of the attempts made from time to time to remove the statutory and other bottlenecks, and strengthen the drug regulatory system in the country.

CHAPTER 3

THE REFORMS THAT WERE NOT TO BE

Previous chapters have brought out that the pharmaceutical industry in India has flourished over decades in the backdrop of the surge in the global demand for medicines and the ability of the Indian pharmaceutical industry to successfully manufacture generic medicines at a much lower cost in comparison to the cost of innovator drugs. However, there are growing concerns with regard to the quality of generic medicines manufactured in India, and details in this regard have been captured in other chapters.[1] Chapter 2 has enumerated the major drawbacks of the existing drug regulatory and other supporting structures.

There can be no doubt that an efficient drug regulatory structure could improve the contribution of the Indian pharmaceutical sector and health outcomes across the globe significantly. The fast-paced developments during the last three decades in the field of medicines, including availability of newer and more sophisticated medical products and increased multilateral trade, especially in case of generics have made the task of drug regulatory authorities increasingly complex. The developments, such as rapid growth of the domestic industry, globalization of the supply chain, the concerns relating to data integrity, complexity arising from the multiplicity of data sources, the massive quantity of data required to be analyzed and development of more potent medical products, underpin the need for a robust regulatory structure. It also highlights the need for induction of talented human resources with specialization in relevant fields and nurturing them through the best training and development programs.

---

[1]. Chapters 1 and 4 may be referred to in this context.

Providence has bestowed India with the capacity to contribute significantly to human health and welfare globally. The COVID-19 pandemic and geo-strategic developments have given India the second opportunity to become the manufacturing hub of quality medicines and medical devices. The concerns expressed globally about the quality of Indian medical products and statements made by authorities of leading importers of generic medicines about diversifying the supply chain of medicines to ensure import of best-quality medicines, are signals that India will need to initiate necessary corrective and preventive action and abhor such methods that might cut the venture short. Not picking up the early warning signals could, in the long run, be disastrous and have a devastating effect on the Indian industry.

In continuation of the details provided in the previous chapter, the present chapter recapitulates the efforts made in the past for reforming drug regulation in India and strengthening drug regulatory structures. The efforts made included those aimed at changing the legal architecture; strengthening of infrastructure; and augmentation of the quality and quantity of resources made available to the drug regulatory structures. These also included efforts aimed at creating more positions in the regulatory structures and improvements in the skill sets through induction, training and development of human resources. The efforts have been only partially successful and remained largely disjointed, and have failed to yield the desired outcomes. Most of the activities that could be accomplished successfully include the amendment in the Drugs & Cosmetics Rules, framing of the Medical Devices Rules, New Drugs & Clinical Trials Rules, strengthening drug testing laboratories, filling up some of the vacant posts and creation of some posts, especially for medical device regulation and drug testing laboratories.

The other achievements of the period were initiation of training programs for regulatory and laboratory staff and establishment of an organization-wide e-governance platform 'Sugam'. The present chapter undertakes an assessment of the efforts made thus far and also throws up areas of concern that need to be addressed.

CENTRALIZATION OF DRUG REGULATION

Big and diverse as India is, adequate provisions need to be made for accommodating regional diversities and aspirations. The federal structure of the Indian polity has given legitimacy to the Indian state, brought about a higher degree of cohesion, and fostered accommodation of different viewpoints, including those of ethnic, cultural, linguistic or religious minorities. There is, however, a need for uniformity and cohesion in some areas, and regulation of medical products is certainly one such area.

Shared or rather diffused responsibility for medical products regulation amongst over three dozen-plus regulators makes regulation in India nebulous. Keeping this in view, the matter regarding centralization of drug regulation has been examined in the past, and a number of committees set up from time to time have made recommendations in this regard. The Pharmaceutical Enquiry Committee, in its report submitted as early as 1954, had underlined the need for centralization of drug regulation in the country. It had suggested that the Drugs Act be amended for centralizing the grant of licenses for manufacturing drugs in the country. However, contrary to the recommendation, the power to grant licenses was entrusted to the state licensing authorities in 1960.

A larger role being entrusted to the central government in the grant of licenses for manufacturing drugs had also been recommended both by the Hathi Committee (1974) and Dr. R. A. Mashelkar Committee (2003). These Committees had highlighted the lack of uniformity and efficiency across the country in implementation of the Drugs & Cosmetics Act, 1940. The Hathi Committee had recommended that the central government should assume responsibility for ensuring statutory enforcement and control over manufacturing of drugs all over the country. The Mashelkar Committee had pointed out that the dual system of drug control had failed to achieve the desired effectiveness and, therefore, the feasibility of bringing all aspects of licensing like loan licensing, certification and complaint handling under the effective control of the Central government should be examined. It had also recommended creation of a Central Drug Administration (CDA) for licensing all manufacturing activities.

In matters concerning regulation of medical products, the federal structure – with the responsibility for regulation being divided between the Centre and the states – has proved to be one of the major weaknesses of the system. Such diffused responsibility has resulted in poor governance of the medical products in India and also restricted the growth of the sector. A strong and globally competitive medical products sector cannot be visualized with decentralized, diffused and amorphous medical products regulatory structures. Action on the reports of the government-appointed committees could have helped in fine-tuning the regulatory processes.

EFFORTS MADE TO STRENGTHEN THE LEGAL FRAMEWORK

In the backdrop of many pitfalls of the current arrangements for drug regulation in India, a number of attempts have been made by the central government to improve drug regulation in the country from time to time, including by proposing changes in the laws and rules. A careful perusal of such efforts indicates that, at best, these were piecemeal and *ad hoc* and did not comprehensively address the pertinent issues that continue to plague the drug regulatory structures and the pharmaceutical industry in India.

The Drugs & Cosmetics (Amendment) Bill, 2003 was one such effort made post 2000. The Bill lapsed with the dissolution of the Lok Sabha (House of People) and the general election in 2004. Another Bill *viz.* the Drugs & Cosmetics (Amendment) Bill, 2005 was introduced after general elections in 2004. The 'Statement of Objects and Reasons' accompanying the Bill stated that the amendments had been proposed to give effect to the recommendations of the expert committee report of 2003. The amendment, however, mainly increased the quantum of punishment for manufacturing spurious and adulterated drugs and the larger issues like fundamental changes to ensure uniformity in drug regulation got overlooked. The amendment resulted in a dichotomy in terms of punishments for manufacturing spurious and adulterated drugs within the country[2] and those imported into the country[3]. This highlights that the entire exercise had been undertaken without due application of mind. The amendments came into force in 2008 and since then, the dichotomy continues on the statue book.

In 2007, another Bill titled the Drugs & Cosmetics (Amendment) Bill, 2007 was introduced in the Parliament. In the 'Statement of Objects & Reasons' of the Bill, it was stated that it sought to centralize drug licensing in India and also proposed to set up a Central Drugs Authority reporting directly to the MoHFW on the lines recommended by the Mashelkar Committee. This Bill was referred to the Parliamentary Standing Committee on Health and Family Welfare for examination. The associations of drug manufacturers, most state drug controllers and state governments, opposed the centralization of drug licensing. The Parliamentary Committee, however, expressed its agreement with the Mashelkar Committee report and endorsed the view that there was an urgent need for establishing a world-class drug regulatory system in the country to effectively handle the health concerns of one-sixth of humanity residing in India and many more in other countries that were using drugs imported from India. The Bill was, however, withdrawn in 2013.

Another Bill *viz.* the Drugs & Cosmetics (Amendment) Bill, 2013 was, thereafter, introduced in the Parliament. The Bill proposed that the CDSCO would be the new Central Drug Authority (CDA). The Bill also proposed that DCG(I) will be the central licensing authority and will be responsible for the day-to-day functioning of the CDA. In the statement accompanying the Bill, it was stated that the revised centralized licensing will cover only seventeen categories of critical drugs included in the proposed Third Schedule to the Bill. The Bill of 2013 thus sought

---

[2.] Section 27 of the Drugs & Cosmetics Act, 1940 prescribes the punishment for manufacture of spurious or adulterated drugs as imprisonment for a period of not less than 10 years and may extend up to imprisonment for life and a fine of not less than Rs. 10 lakh or three times the value of drugs confiscated, whichever is more.

[3.] Section 13 of the Drugs & Cosmetics Act, 1940 prescribes the punishment for import of spurious or adulterated drugs as imprisonment, which may extend up to three years and a fine up to Rs. 5000.

to confine the scope of centralized licensing for manufacturing, sale and export to seventeen categories of drugs manufactured in the country. It had, however, proposed to empower the Central Government to amend the Third Schedule to expand the number of drugs that would be subject to centralized licensing. The export of drugs was proposed to be brought within the domain of the central licensing authority.

Falling short of the recommendations of experts, the Bill sought to introduce another set of dual system for grant of licenses. This Bill too was referred to the Department Related Parliamentary Standing Committee on Health. Several provisions of the Bill were opposed by the pharmaceutical industry and many state governments. Even the Ministry of Commerce opposed the provision relating to the introduction of an additional layer for regulating exports. The primary objection of the states and the pharmaceutical associations was with regard to introduction of central licensing. The states were apprehensive of losing the authority and the pharmaceutical associations feared more stringent regulatory controls.

The Standing Committee also recommended that the decision to place *Betalactums* and *Cephalosporins* antibiotics and parenteral preparations in the Third Schedule, which would have included drugs reserved for central licensing, may be looked at *de novo*. The Standing Committee also recommended doing away with the proposed CDA as it would be too large and unwieldy. The Confederation of small and medium pharmaceutical enterprises (SME) expressed the apprehension that centralization of drug licensing would kill the SME pharmaceutical units and further strengthen the already powerful multinational companies by increasing the compliance cost.

While the Drugs & Cosmetics (Amendment) Bill, 2013 was still pending in the Parliament, the MoHFW invited comments on a new Drugs & Cosmetics (Amendment) Bill, 2015. This new version of the Bill had incorporated several changes recommended by the Standing Committee of the Parliament. With a view to ensuring clarity, FDCs were specifically proposed to be included in the Third Schedule of the proposed Bill.

Based on extensive consultations with all stakeholders, the Bill for amending the Drugs & Cosmetics Act was further revised by the MoHFW.

The revised Bill, finalized after detailed consultations with all stakeholders, sought to remove a large number of concerns in the existing law, including those relating to removal of different punishments for import of adulterated or spurious drugs and their manufacture within the country. However, it was far from what had been recommended by various committees, i.e., to establish a single regulatory mechanism for drugs in the country.

When that Bill was to be placed before the Cabinet, the PMO decided that it may, in the first instance, be examined by a Group of Ministers (GoM). After a very brief discussion in the very first meeting of the GoM chaired by the then Finance Minister, Arun Jaitley, it was decided that keeping in view the large-scale changes proposed in the Act, it would be appropriate that a completely new Bill is prepared to replace the existing law. It was also decided that, for the time being, separate rules be carved out for regulating medical devices under the existing Drugs & Cosmetics Act, 1940. In the process, the most important challenge that still remains unaddressed is the enactment of a suitable parliamentary legislation that takes into account the constitutional provisions and balances the need for ushering in much desired legal reforms in the field of medical products regulation.

SOME FORWARD MOVEMENT

Following the decision of the GoM, the MoHFW carried out elaborate consultations with all stakeholders for drafting rules for the regulation of medical devices. In addition to that, two separate Bills – one each concerning Drugs & Cosmetics and the medical devices – were prepared in 2016 and placed before the then Minister of Health and Family Welfare for *in principle* approval before public consultations were undertaken. However, the draft Bills never came back from the Minister.

The public/stakeholders consultations in respect of Medical Device Rules saw unprecedented response from the national and international bodies, manufacturers and consumer associations, think tanks, universities, individual medical device manufacturers, state governments, clinicians, etc. In addition to the written comments and suggestions, meetings were also arranged on working days and almost on all Saturdays and Sundays for a few months in which officers of the CDSCO, representatives of industry, consumer associations, academic institutions and even representatives of the World Health Organization participated in large numbers. Academicians from outside the country also participated in these deliberations.

There were differences on some issues amongst different industry associations, and also between the industry and the CDSCO officials. However, notwithstanding their initial reservations, eventually everyone agreed on the proposed course of action. What was clear from the meetings with stakeholders was that every participant, irrespective of the organizational affiliations, was keen on using the opportunity to be part of the mission to create a world-class regulatory structure for medical products in India.

Each provision in the proposed rules was read and discussed threadbare. The camaraderie exhibited by everyone was unprecedented. At the end of this elaborate exercise, medical devices rules were finalized in conformity with the Global Harmonization Task Force (GHTF) framework and best international practices. The rules were notified on January 31, 2017.

Considering the difficulties in taking the new Bills to a logical conclusion, the time required for completion of the parliamentary processes and the need for a transition to the new regime, other *ad interim* measures were initiated and implemented in a mission mode to improve regulation of medical products in the country. The short-term solutions evolved and implemented took note of the problems that had been identified in the reports of the parliamentary committees, representations made by various organizations and individuals to the parliamentary committees and to the government, interaction with a large number of stake-holders, etc., and comprised a large number of steps that could have been taken without amending the law.

An elaborate exercise was also initiated for carving out separate rules for regulating New Drugs and Clinical Trials; manufacturing and import of drugs into the country; regulation of sale and marketing of drugs, including e-Pharmacy and Cosmetics rules.

In the case of sale of drugs, it was proposed to make it mandatory to share information regarding purchase, sale and dispensing of drugs on the online portal by manufacturers, the brick-and-mortar pharmacies and the e-pharmacies. This was considered necessary to enable tracking of each drug unit from the manufacturing plant to the consumer. The proposal had initially been placed in the public domain as a concept note in 2015. During the oral discussions held in the MoHFW, the representatives of both the e-pharmacies and the brick-and-mortar pharmacies had agreed on the broad contours of the proposal, but both of them raised a number of objections when the concept note was made public. Both sets of pharmacies were clearly not keen on being regulated and held accountable.

The drafts of all the rules referred to above, had been prepared for public consultation during 2016 and early 2017, and these were in various stages of approvals or vetting by the Legislative Department in June 2017. Some of these rules have since been finalized. All others are still pending. Earlier, as an interim measure, the Drugs & Cosmetics Rules, 1945 was amended to ensure compliance with best practices till the new set of rules could be notified. These included amendments in rules concerning clinical trials, mandatory stability tests, bioequivalence and bioavailability studies, and joint inspection of manufacturing units before production, and issuance of perpetual licenses for drugs unless the licenses were suspended or cancelled by the Licensing Authority. Unfortunately, the pace of work relating to refining the law and rules for drug regulation were put on the backburner after June 2017 with the changes in the senior management in the MoHFW.

As such, most of the efforts made to improve the legislative framework were, at best, *ad hoc* and not thought through. There can be no doubt that the pre-independence legislation *viz.* The Drugs & Cosmetics Act, 1940 should have been consigned to history a long time back. It is a matter of great concern that even after seven and a half decades of India's independence, a new law to regulate medical products in the country has not been enacted and the archaic law that has outlived its utility still continues to be stretched. The fact that regulation of medical products marketed in the country and also those exported to other countries can be treated with such disdain, paints the so-called pharmacy of the world poorly. What compounds the situation further is the fact that there is still inadequate appreciation of such fault-lines, and the authorities at the state level continue to be vested with more roles. The question that needs to be addressed under these circumstances is how can impeccable quality of medical products be ensured in a poorly-regulated market like India?

THE GRAND PLAN AND ITS SCALING DOWN

Taking into account the importance of the sector, the first major effort for up-gradation of the drug regulatory infrastructure and addition of human resources was initiated in 2012 as a grandiose plan proposing an expenditure of over Rs. 6000 crore during the 12th Five Year Plan (2012–17). It proposed augmentation of the drug regulatory system, including manpower and infrastructure both at the central and state levels. Owing to the disconnect between the different departments of the Government of India, there were no takers for the scheme outside the MoHFW, and the matter continued to linger for quite some time. The plan was subsequently scaled down and appraised in two meetings of the Expenditure Finance Committee (EFC)[4] headed by Secretary, Department of Expenditure during the first quarter of 2014. A truncated version of the scheme was recommended by the EFC at a budgetary allocation of Rs. 1750 crore. Out of this, Rs. 900 crore was proposed for the central structures and Rs. 850 crore for the states.

In July 2014, this was one of the pending issues. After a fresh perusal of the papers relating to the scheme, it was pointed out that it might not be feasible to implement all components that had been included in the scheme as these would have required prior planning and preparatory action along with the cooperation of the state governments, and a part of the 12th Five-Year Plan was already over. Nevertheless, a number of activities appeared

---

[4]. EFC is a forum for appraisal of proposals where the outcomes are not capable of being measured in quantifiable terms. It is serviced by the Department of Expenditure.

to be doable. It was, however, considered that even if 50% of the activities, especially those related to strengthening and re-equipping of drug testing laboratories and addition of some manpower could be achieved, it would be worth its while because starting all over again would have meant a loss of a few more years.

DISCUSSIONS IN PMO AND CCEA APPROVAL

Based on the EFC recommendations, the proposal was circulated for soliciting the views of the Ministries/Departments concerned of the central government and all states/union territories(UTs). There was an overwhelming support for the scheme. Most of the states pointed out that more resources should be allocated to the states as compared with the central structures. Based on inter-ministerial consultations and consultations with states and union territories, towards the end of November 2014, the final Note was sent to the Cabinet Secretariat for placing it before the Cabinet Committee on Economic Affairs (CCEA)[5] for approval.

The proposal got stuck in the PMO where a view was expressed that the role of the central government in regulation of drugs ought to be minimized and the role of states increased. It was also considered that an outlay of Rs. 1750 crore was on the higher side and states should fend for themselves. However, after two rounds of discussions in the PMO, it was decided that the MoHFW will have a fresh look at the proposal and then make a presentation in the PMO. The PMO officials also indicated that this will provide an opportunity to the new Secretary to apply himself to the issues at hand independently. After a series of discussions within the Ministry and further presentation in the PMO, the matter was finally approved by the CCEA in August 2015.

[5.] CCEA is a standing Committee of the Cabinet and is constituted as per the provisions of the Government of India (Transaction of Business) Rules, 1961. All proposals having a bearing on the economy of the country, including projects and schemes beyond a specified threshold measured in monetary terms, are required to be placed before this Committee for approval.

COMPONENTS OF SCHEMES

The central sector scheme, as approved by CCEA, envisaged setting up of six new drug testing laboratories[6]; eight minilabs at air and seaports; augmentation of facilities in the existing seven drug testing laboratories of the CDSCO, duly equipped with the state-of-the art testing equipment/ machines and additional manpower; setting up of a training academy for drug regulators; construction of new office buildings; and creation of an e-Governance mechanism for electronic handling of the entire work entrusted to the CDSCO, along with networking of the CDSCO and state regulators. It also envisaged creation of 2500 additional posts of laboratory and regulatory officials as part of the CDSCO strengthening.

As far as states were concerned, the approval accorded proposed the setting up of ten new drug testing laboratories; augmentation of facilities at the existing 31 drug testing laboratories in various states; commissioning of 20 mobile drug testing laboratories and creation of 3000 additional regulatory and laboratory posts in different states.

The mechanism for transfer of funds to the states/UTs was to be decided by the MoHFW. Given the history of the proposal, the MoHFW was not sure whether the scheme will get approval of the CCEA at all or if the proposal will get blocked again. Keeping this in view, except sounding the state governments about the possibility of its approval, no concrete action had been taken for execution of the scheme. It was only after the approval of the CCEA that action was initiated for implementing both the central and state components; however, obtaining approval was easier and its implementation, including locating the required money and creation of additional posts, proved to be a Herculean task.

In the month of August 2015, all state governments were requested to sign a memorandum of understanding and also send their proposals in the format prepared for release of funds against specific items that formed part of the scheme. In addition to *demi official* letters sent through speed post,

---

[6.] Drugs as defined in the Drugs & Cosmetics Act, 1940 include medical devices. Two of the laboratories proposed to be set up were for medical device testing.

the communication was also sent through e-mail and the officials concerned were also informed telephonically. Separately, states were also requested to provide land free of cost for establishing central drug testing laboratories and the CDSCO offices. All port authorities were also requested to provide space for minilabs. Directions were also issued to all the CDSCO zonal/sub-zonal heads to locate land for laboratories and offices. For facilitating the transfer of funds to the states, a formula based on a weighted average of the number of manufacturing units in the state, its population and the number of licensed sales outlets of chemists in the state concerned was evolved.

THE ROAD BLOCK

For the benefit of those who are not familiar with the working of the governmental system in India, it must be clarified that obtaining approval of the Cabinet or its committees is not sufficient for implementing a scheme in India, and it is only the beginning. The budgetary allocations for the sector are decided by the Ministry of Finance each year on the basis of projections made by the Ministry/Department concerned. Invariably, the allocations fall far short of the funds required for implementation of any scheme. Further, the Department of Expenditure has the final say as far as creation of posts is concerned and even after creation of posts, filling them up takes years depending on the efficiency of the recruiting agency, whether it is the Union Public Service Commission or the Staff Selection Commission. Also, it is necessary that the states are on board as actual implementation is dependent on their cooperation.

Despite very strong recommendations of the MoHFW year after year, the Ministry of Finance could not locate sufficient funds for the scheme at the time of finalization of budgetary proposals for presentation to the Parliament. Further, the restrictions on the outflow of funds during a quarter did not permit more than a fixed percentage of the allocated funds to be spent even from out of the allocated budget. Luckily, some funds could be located for the scheme towards the end of the Financial Year 2015–16 and 2016–17 from the funds allocated for the National Health

Mission, which also included strengthening of drug regulatory structures as one of its components. Despite regular follow up, including discussions with senior officials of the state concerned, many states did not come forward to avail the central assistance.

STRENGTHENING OF CENTRAL STRUCTURES

In case of the central component, a series of proactive steps were initiated to implement the activities included in the scheme. One of the weakest areas at that point of time was the drugs testing laboratories, which had no state-of-the-art equipment and, in most cases, the required manpower was not available, as detailed in the previous chapter. A committee of Directors of the drug testing laboratories visited each laboratory and firmed up the requirements for machinery and equipment required in each laboratory. This work was also accorded high priority as it had also been decided that all samples of drugs collected as part of the drug survey 2014-16 will be tested only in government laboratories.[7]

Based on the recommendations of that committee of Directors, orders were placed within a month of the approval accorded by the CCEA for procuring equipment like High performance liquid chromatography (HPLC) machines, etc. Each drug testing laboratory was also permitted to engage 30 qualified staff on contract basis for test and analysis of the samples of drugs. Further, the Directors of the laboratories were asked to take immediate steps for getting their respective laboratories inspected, accredited and certified, and have the equipment that was non-functional repaired or replaced. It was made clear that the laboratories that had not been accredited will not be allowed to function after a specified date. Subsequently, the Drugs & Cosmetics Rules, 1945 were also amended to make certification/accreditation of drug testing laboratories mandatory.

The state-of-the-art equipment and additional contractual manpower were provided to laboratories in time for them to take up the testing and

---

[7.] See Chapter 5 for details.

analysis of the samples picked up as part of the national survey. With the change in focus, all central drug testing laboratories were NABL- accredited and ISO-certified within a year and a half. Steps were also taken for filling up the existing vacancies in a mission mode.

Separately, humongous efforts were made for locating land for the CDSCO offices and laboratories. However, the response of many states was lukewarm. The Government of Himachal Pradesh provided a piece of land at Baddi in Solan district for the sub-zonal office of the CDSCO and the Government of Odisha provided land at Bhubaneshwar for setting up a drug testing laboratory. In case of Madhya Pradesh, a parcel of land available with the Central Public Works Department was located in Indore, and the process was initiated for its transfer for setting up the zonal office and drug testing laboratory.

A parcel of land where medicines for distribution to health facilities of the government were stored in tin sheds by the Medical Stores Organization (MSO) under the MoHFW was identified in South Delhi. In Patna, built-up space was offered in old AIIMS campus in 2017 as the state government did not respond even after the matter had been taken up with the Chief Minister. In Chennai, a piece of land belonging to the MSO was identified for construction of the zonal office of the CDSCO. It was decided to locate the training academy for drug regulators within the campus of the National Institute of Biologicals, Noida on a vacant portion of the land without disturbing the ambience or the functionality of the rest of the Institute.

Things were moving in the right direction. However, when designs had been frozen, the then DGHS started raising issues in case of the South Delhi and Chennai plots, demanding that half of the constructed area be given to the MSO for its use. The issue was discussed in a meeting arranged at the level of Secretary, MoHFW. Though an agreement was reached on the constructed area to be apportioned between two organizations, i.e., the CDSCO and MSO, the then DGHS again raised fresh issues after a month. It was clear by this time that the project will continue to be stalled on one pretext or the other.

The Municipal Corporation of Delhi (North) had also offered one of the hospital sites for setting up the training academy and the medical devices testing laboratory. However, since the cost of land was very high, it was decided that some spare land available at the Indian Pharmacopoeia Commission, Ghaziabad will be used for setting up the medical devices testing laboratory. In case of the Chennai project, after a lot of persuasion, the land was made available to the CDSCO for housing the zonal office.

After the design of the training academy building within the NIB premises had been frozen, the then Additional Secretary in the MoHFW raised doubts about its feasibility. There were also issues with the non-availability of funds and, therefore, the plan to have a separate building for the training academy had to be dropped. After discussions, Director, NIB offered the Ground Floor of the building housing the Library of the Institute as the venue for imparting training to drug regulatory officials. The NIB also offered the conference room and other facilities available in the NIB, including the hostel for training purposes, subject to availability on *ad hoc* basis.

With a lot of pushing around, the projects at different places started to move forward. Towards the middle of 2020, the projects at Baddi, Chennai, Bhubaneshwar and Indore had been completed. Due to non-availability of manpower and equipment, the facilities remain unutilized even at the time of publication of this book in 2021. The project at Ghaziabad for medical devices testing laboratory remains stuck as the contractor has reportedly abandoned the work. The laboratory project at Patna was not pursued after June 2017. In short, the projects that would have been completed by or before the Financial Year 2019–20 are still languishing with no manpower in place and no equipment. The tragedy is that adequate manpower for the drug testing laboratory at Hyderabad has not been sanctioned as yet, though this laboratory came into existence a decade and a half back.[8]

[8.] Two posts of Deputy Directors for Drug Testing Laboratories were sanctioned in 2016. One of these two posts was earmarked for the laboratory at Hyderabad. However, these could not be filled up till 2021.

INADEQUATE HUMAN RESORUCES

The total requirement of the drug regulatory staff to handle the responsibility currently entrusted to the CDSCO is around 4500 personnel, with 2800 on regulatory side and 1700 on laboratory side. At present, the total strength of the organization is pegged at below 700 for both the regulatory and laboratory staff. Further, a large number of posts in the organization, including those in drug testing laboratories, have fallen vacant and could not be filled up.

Based on the approval accorded by the CCEA and to make up the deficiency in a staggered manner, the Department of Expenditure was approached to create additional posts in 2015–16. Around 50 odd posts were agreed to be created after two detailed rounds of formal queries and a discussion against 2500 approved by the CCEA and around 750 proposed by the MoHFW in the first phase.

UPGRADATION OF THE CDSCO AS AN ATTACHED OFFICE

Bureaucrats, in general, are very particular about their entitlements in terms of timely promotions, perquisites and other benefits due to them. Any delay in their promotion is invariably not acceptable to them. Even if there are no sanctioned posts, the lower posts stand upgraded *post haste* to ensure their timely promotion. Bureaucracy, however, does not think of any such solutions in so far as implementation of projects is concerned. It also does not permit any organization other than the one headed by a bureaucrat to flourish.

Bureaucrats believe that higher positions in the government are the prerogative of only those who are members of particular services. A case relating to up-gradation of the post of DCG(I) illustrates this aspect. Based on a proposal floated by the MoHFW, the Union Cabinet had, in January 2007, approved that the post of the DCG(I) be upgraded to the level of Additional Secretary to the Government of India, pending amendment of the Drugs & Cosmetics Act, 1940 for setting up the Central Drug

Authority. However, the approval of the Cabinet was never implemented and the post continues to be operated at the level of Joint Secretary to the Government of India. What is more worrisome is that it continued to be manned on *ad hoc* basis as an additional charge for five years. Of course, this was amongst others facilitated by a court case filed in the Madras High Court that remained *sub judice* for a number of years. The Central Drug Authority is also nowhere on the horizon.

The CDSCO still continues to be the subordinate office[9] of the DGHS and, technically, all its proposals have to be moved through the DGHS. The DGHS also continues to give directions to the CDSCO even in operational matters. The national regulator does not enjoy any autonomy in its functioning. The proposal for up gradation of the CDSCO as an Attached Office[10] of the MoHFW had been discussed many times over the last two decades based on the recommendations of many committees that had been set up in the past. However, it did not go beyond discussion.

A proposal based on Satyananda Mishra[11] Committee Report was processed in 2015 and a draft Cabinet Note for creation of different verticals for regulating different products was prepared for inter-ministerial consultation. It also proposed to make the CDSCO an attached office of the MoHFW; up gradation of the post of DCG(I) to HAG+ level; and creation

---

[9.] Subordinate Offices generally function as field establishments or as agencies responsible for the detailed execution of the policies of the government. They function under the direction of an attached office, or where the volume of executive direction involved is not considerable, directly under a department. In the latter case, they assist the Departments concerned in handling executive and technical matters in their respective fields of specialization.

[10.] Attached Offices provide detailed executive directions required in the implementation of the policies, as laid down from time to time by the Ministry/Department to which they are attached. They also serve as a repository of information and also advise the department on various aspects of matter dealt by them.

[11.] Satyananda Mishra was the Secretary in the Department of Personnel & Training and also held the post of Chief Information Commissioner. The other eminent members of the committee were Dr. M K Bhan and Professor (Dr) Ranjit Roy Chaudhury. Dr. Bhan had worked in various capacities, including that of the Secretary, Department of Biotechnology. He transformed India's biotech program and set up a number of institutions, enabling industry–academia collaboration in the field. Professor Ranjit Roy Chaudhury was a leading medical researcher, a specialist in medical teaching and a health planner for the country. He had chaired various committees, including the one on the clinical trials.

of six posts of Additional Drug Controller Generals for heading different verticals; and setting up a national academy for training drug regulators. Each of these verticals was to be manned by an officer from the relevant specializations *viz.* Drugs; Medical Devices; Biologicals & other Emerging areas; Quality Control and Laboratories; and *AYUSH* drugs respectively.

The recommendations were balanced and pragmatic. In the meantime, the CDSCO had also been identified as one of the organizations for introduction of Human Resources Management System (HRMS) as part of an initiative borrowed from Gujarat. The objective of the exercise was to enhance organizational efficiency through induction, retention and development of high-quality human resources. A brief note on the subject was shared with the Department of Personnel & Training with the approval of the then Secretary, MoHFW. However, the senior officials of MoHFW subsequently ensured that the proposal did not materialize even after it had been approved by the Minister of Health and Family Welfare.

The issue was further discussed in a presentation made in the conference room of the Minister of Health and Family Welfare. After detailed discussions, the Minister had directed that the new Secretary may go through the proposal again before the matter was processed further. That was the end of the proposal. However, the issue of strengthening the CDSCO continues to be discussed and deliberated, including at the level of Cabinet Secretary whenever there is a crisis.

VACANT POSITIONS IN THE CDSCO

An important impediment in the smooth functioning of the CDSCO is a large number of vacancies in various grades. In July 2014, nearly 60% of the 575 odd sanctioned posts in the CDSCO were vacant. With a lot of effort, including discussions with the officials in the Union Public Service Commission and regular pursuance of the matter with the Staff Selection Commission, over 300 vacant posts were filled up during 2014–2017. Most of the posts that could not be filled up at that point of time remain vacant even in 2021. In the interregnum, many more posts have fallen vacant.

To overcome the difficulties in the recruitment process, the recruitment rules for all posts in drug testing laboratories were taken up for revision in 2016 and a series of meetings were arranged in the Ministry. The matter was later referred to two different committees. The result is that the Recruitment Rules (RRs) have not been amended and in the absence of revision having taken place, the filling up of vacancies has not been feasible and many posts have lapsed. The MoHFW has, in 2021 reportedly, started exploring the possibility of reviving the lapsed posts.

TRAINING AND DEVELOPMENT OF HUMAN RESOURCES

The complexity of the subject coupled with the fact that most of the drug regulatory personnel join with inadequate or no prior experience and there are hardly any courses on drug regulatory practices in most Indian universities, good training programs for regulators are indispensable. Even for those who have worked in the industry earlier or have been working in drug regulatory structures, enhancement of their skill sets and familiarization with the new developments is necessary for comprehending the latest scientific innovations, international regulatory practices that continue to evolve and other developments. This is all the more important in the Indian context, given the role played by the Indian pharmaceutical industry in making affordable medicines available globally.

The training and developmental activities in case of drug regulators, including laboratory staff, have always been given a very low priority in India. Till 2015, there were no structured programs for imparting training to drug regulatory officials. In fact, the matter was not considered important enough to engage the attention of the government. As a result, there was no uniformity in regulatory practices across states. The officials learned largely from their exposure to the work and generally picked up the wrong practices and shortcuts that compromised quality.

It was in the above background that during 2015–2017, a number of training activities for the drug enforcement and laboratory staff of the central and the state governments were started by adopting the field and forum approach – combining traditional classroom training with on-the-job training supervised by competent resource persons. These included training programs organized in-house; in association with the industry; at the Indian Pharmacopoeia Commission; in association with drug regulators of other countries and the WHO. The basic objective of these training programs was to build the capacity of drug regulatory officials across the country with a view to to ensuring. Uniform implementation of the law and removing knowledge barriers. Combined training programs were conducted for both regulatory and laboratory officials from the Centre and the states to enable them to understand each other's perspective. These also sought to address the concerns relating to competence of the regulatory and laboratory officials in enforcement of law.

In addition to a large number of workshops organized for the CDSCO and state drug regulatory officials, 10 different training programs – ranging from induction to advanced levels – were organized between October 2015 to May 2017, in which around 700 drug regulatory and laboratory officials from the CDSCO and states were trained. Several capacity-building activities, including basic as well as advanced workshops on Good Manufacturing Practices (GMP) and inspections were arranged in coordination with the WHO. A training program to enhance the skills of laboratory personnel of the central and state governments was started at the Indian Pharmacopoeia Commission, Ghaziabad. One training program was conducted every month for the laboratory officials.

It has, however, been pointed out that the training programs organized between 2015 and 2017 were short-term measures essentially aimed at addressing the shortcomings perceived in terms of the capacity of regulatory and laboratory officials of the drug control departments at the Centre and the states. These were, however, *ad hoc* one-time efforts to bridge the perceived gaps in the knowledge of officials. Initially, there were doubts about the participation of officials from states in such training programs given the sense of sub-nationalism and deep territorialism sparred amongst others by competition between states for garnering investments in the pharmaceutical sector and different political parties being in power in the centre and the states. It was a pleasant surprise that most states spared their officials for the training programs.

It was for the first time that barriers between the central and state regulators on the one hand and laboratory and regulatory officials on the other hand were sought to be dismantled. This enabled them to share the practices followed in their respective states and laboratories with each other and also with resource persons. These programs could, however, not take into account the long-term requirements of augmenting the capacity of structures as a whole.

Drug Inspectors, analysts and other regulatory staff must constantly update their knowledge about evolving regulatory developments, scientific techniques, investigation processes, etc. These require different kinds of training toolkits and methodologies. While formulating organizational training and developmental plans, clarity about the competencies, awareness and skill sets needed at different levels is important. An exercise had been started in 2016 for devising training programs for crosscutting functional capacities needed for formulation, implementation and reviewing strategies, programs and projects for senior management and capacities associated with the thematic areas for officials at middle and supervisory management levels to ensure smoother communication with the clients for ensuring meaningful outcomes. The cultural shifts and changes in attitude, practices and behavior of individuals, groups and organizations were also sought to be integrated with the training and developmental activities. However, the exercise was abandoned after 2017 and even the existing training programs were discontinued. No long-term plan could be evolved and the proposal to set up the National Academy for Drug Regulators has been buried.

E-GOVERNANCE FOR BETTER RECORD MANAGEMENT

The previous chapter, *inter alia*, brought out concerns with regard to the management of records in the CDSCO. The then Additional Secretary, R.K. Jain and Secretary, Health and Family Welfare, Lov Verma, approved the launch of a two-pronged strategy for digitalization of the CDSCO processes in early 2015. As a short-term measure, the development of the software for handling clinical trial-related processes was entrusted to the National Informatics Centre (NIC). The software was developed by NIC in 15 months. However, it was noted that the software could not handle the heavy workload.

A larger project for the development of the software to handle organization-wide activities in the CDSCO electronically was awarded to C-DAC. C-DAC was also asked to integrate the NIC software with C-DAC solutions. The development of the new software was taken up in phases, and the first phase included only the activities undertaken at the CDSCO. It was to be expanded in later phases to the states. Eventually, it envisaged to accomplish the online processing of all applications at the CDSCO headquarters as well as other offices, laboratories and state drug regulatory authorities.

The e-Governance system developed by C-DAC was christened '*SUGAM*' – literally meaning 'ease'. Activities relating to import registration and licensing of drugs and medical devices; registration of cosmetics; registration of ethics committees;[12] permission to conduct clinical trials and bioavailability and bioequivalence studies; permitting import of drugs by individual patients for personal use; grant of test license for import of small quantities of drugs for test and analysis are now being handled through *SUGAM*. Online processing of protocols at CDL, Kasauli had also been integrated with *SUGAM* and the customs online system '*ICEGATE*' to ensure seamless clearing of imported consignments of drugs at all the CDSCO port offices.

SUGAM had, in view of its efficiency, been awarded the Computer Society of India Nihilent e-Governance Award of Excellence, 2016. Though *SUGAM* has been in operation for quite some time now, the job is still half done. There are still issues with the software; it still does not cover activities

---

12. Ethics committee is an independent body comprising medical professionals and non-medical members, including laymen. The Committee is responsible for verifying that the safety, integrity and human rights of subjects participating in a particular clinical trial are protected. It provides public reassurance that the ethical principles are observed in clinical trials.

undertaken by state regulators; and data relating to inspections, violations of law, substandard drugs and their recall, etc., are still not available through *SUGAM*. The software will require up gradation, strengthening and expansion to realize the full potential of information technology in consonance with the Digital India initiative.

STRENGTHENING OF IPC AND NIB

Despite approvals from the government and the availability of necessary resources, the setting up of the state-of-the-art laboratory at the Indian Pharmacopoeia Commission has been on hold as the contractor has left the work unfinished and the authorities have not been able to take a decision to engage another contractor to complete the work. In the process, the investment made is getting wasted. It needs to be recognized that the mismatch between the structures, human resources and equipment blocks the scarce resources and in a resource starved country, any such mismatch is criminal.

As far as the NIB is concerned, with a little augmentation of its facilities, it could help the bio-tech innovators and industry by providing support required in terms of technical frameworks for enhancing the quality and productivity; take up the responsibility for training the manpower to make them industry ready and develop human resources for quality control of biologicals; fill the gap in the area of academics and high-end research by opening its facilities to students and industry professionals; and engage with scientific research and technological developments by establishing linkages with different institutions in India and abroad.

Eventually, the NIB could assist the bio-tech entrepreneurs in navigating the international markets and establish world-class healthcare organizations. The institute could become the go-to place for the industry, academic institutions, etc., in case any guidance or technical support is required. This will, besides ensuring uniformity, also cut down costs for the industry and help NIB to eventually become self-financing.

Between 2014 and 2017, the NIB had made some progress in furtherance of its activities. A number of reputed international organizations had proposed to collaborate with the NIB. A majority of its laboratories had been accredited as per ISO 17025: 2005 by NABL and eight of them have been functioning as the Central Drugs Laboratories (CDL) from 15.03.2017 onwards. From 2015 onwards, the NIB has also started training programs for students from North Eastern and hilly states.

An Institutional Development Plan (IDP) spanning five years (2017–2022) for strengthening both the training activities for development of highly skilled manpower and augmenting R&D activities at NIB had been prepared under the guidance of a committee of experts. It included manpower augmentation, creation of central instrumentation facility and strengthening of Bioinformatics Division. The plan was expected to expand the NIB's expertise relating to biological processes and provide a robust scientific base to review the new and pipeline biologicals, besides reviewing new indications for already-approved products. The above initiative has, however, remained on paper and the IDP, which was to be implemented by March 2022, is yet to be considered and approved in August 2021. The excellent infrastructural facilities at the NIB are, in the process, being used sub-optimally.

To sum up, the problem with the regulation of medical products in India reflects the lack of ownership and sincerity of purpose, both at the political executive and the senior bureaucratic levels. Strengthening the medical products regulatory structures has not been accorded the requisite priority and even when some efforts were made, these did not succeed for want of resources, commitment and ownership. The non-availability of resources in sufficient measure over the years for the health sector in general, and medical products regulation and promotion of medical products industry in particular, has led to a situation where the urgent and immediate health concerns continue to usurp most of the allocated resources, leaving very little for the long-term structural reforms. Hence, only sporadic and incremental improvements in drug regulatory structures in India have been possible. The larger issues concerning responsibility and accountability of structures in terms of the constitutional and legislative remit have remained unaddressed.

Restructuring and reformation of any existing structure is a long, grueling and arduous journey, spanning years. The journey becomes much more meandering when such restructuring affects the entrenched and vested interests and more specifically, when there is a lack of ownership at governmental levels. Restructuring organizations dealing with medical products regulation in India is no exception with serious objections from associations of manufacturers, state governments and even associations of chemists and druggists with strong political connections.

The restructuring of India's drug regulatory machinery will have to be more like a passage to a new way of life and not just an altered way of regulation. It will require meticulous planning and execution with continuity in leadership and a strong sense of ownership and commitment at the highest levels. This is especially so as most of the stakeholders are comfortable with the *status quo* that provides them with an escape route from being held accountable. The so-called pharmacy of the world can no longer afford the luxury of having a flawed legislative framework and a lax and diffused regulatory structure, and it is time for necessary corrective steps to be initiated.

CHAPTER 4

QUALITY OF INDIAN MEDICAL PRODUCTS

MEDICAL PRODUCTS AND HEALTHCARE DELIVERY

The efficiency of any healthcare system is dependent on a host of factors, including the quality of medical products, good hospital infrastructure, trained human resources, their skill-sets and the overall level of hygiene in the society. Of all these factors, the quality, safety and efficacy of medical products, to a large extent, is determined by players and factors substantially beyond the control of the establishment delivering healthcare services.

The developments in the field of medical science have facilitated precision in the delivery of healthcare. Be it the prevention, diagnosis, treatment, cure or management of diseases, the scientific developments have made the tasks simpler and results more predictable. At the same time, given the potency of modern medicines, a bad quality medical product can cause unprecedented harm not only to the individual patient who is administered the medicine but also the public at large, including by giving rise to antimicrobial resistance.[1] In this background, it is imperative that the medical products are of the best possible quality and are not compromised.

This chapter looks at issues relating to the quality of medical products and includes the findings of the largest ever drug survey undertaken anywhere in the world for determining the quality of drugs marketed in India; risk-based inspections of pharmaceutical manufacturing units undertaken during 2016–17; and the findings of surprise inspections of bulk storage facilities in Delhi in 2017. This has been supplemented by

---

[1] The examples of Heparin detailed in Chapter 9 may be referred to.

the author's personal experience in a key position in the MoHFW that included handling drug regulation.

UNDERSTANDING THE QUALITY OF MEDICAL PRODUCTS

Borrowing from the definition of quality in other disciplines, 'quality' in the context of medical products can be construed to imply a state of being free from defects, deficiencies and any significant variations from specifications achieved through a complete conformance with certain standards resulting in the uniformity of a product and its ability to deliver the intended results consistently during its shelf life. A quality drug should meet the safety, potency, efficacy, stability-related requirements, and should have been manufactured by observing all required processes.

Quality by design is premised on the logic that most quality crises and problems relate to the way in which a product had been designed in the first place.[2] Keeping in view the fact that any defect in the product design or in the manufacturing process of a medical product cannot be rectified at a later stage, quality has to be designed into a product and the manufacturing processes. Quality by design was also the central issue in the International Conference on Harmonization of Technical Requirements for Registration of Pharmaceuticals for Human Use.[3]

Quality assurance activities are preventive in nature and are intended to monitor the processes followed to manage and create deliverables, and verify that the processes have been followed. This builds the trust between different stakeholders, such as the management, customers, government agencies, regulators and third parties, about the quality requirements having been met at various stages. Quality Control is a reactive process and is aimed at detecting issues with conformance, and it monitors and verifies

---

[2.] https://www.ncbi.nlm.nih.gov/pmc/articles/PMC4070262/#:~:text=Quality%20by%20design% 0(QbD)%20is,designed%20in%20the%20first%20place.

[3.] International Conference on Harmonization of Technical Requirements for Registration of Pharmaceuticals for Human Use brings together the regulatory authorities of Europe, Japan and the United States, and experts from the pharmaceutical industry in the three regions to discuss scientific and technical aspects of product registration.

that the deliverables meet the defined quality standards. It ensures that materials utilized to manufacture a pharmaceutical product and the end products meet the specifications relating to identity, strength, purity and other characteristics.

The quality of medicines needs to be built-into the design and verified on a continuous basis throughout the process, in addition to certification through end product testing and analysis. Relying exclusively on end product testing and analysis would be insufficient to ensure quality, safety and efficacy of medicines or detecting impurities or other problems with the quality of drugs that could arise due to faulty processes or even problems with the raw materials.

Most government officials, the regulators and a large segment of pharmaceutical manufacturers in India hold the view that while theoretically the entire process – starting with raw materials to finished formulations and product quality – is important, it would suffice if the end product met the qualitative requirements through the processes of testing and analysis. The Indian narrative does not accord much importance to adherence with prescribed processes. It has also largely been ignoring the quality of raw materials or the API/KSM/DI used for manufacturing. To buttress any objection, it is often argued that the modern sophisticated machines are capable of identifying any quality compromises during test and analysis and if a product passed all stipulated tests, its quality should not be doubted.

Some associations of domestic pharmaceutical manufacturers argue that the excessive emphasis by drug regulators of many advanced countries on process quality and related aspects is misplaced perfectionism and is not worth the time, money and effort required to be invested on those aspects. They assert that perfectionism in the processes cannot be the ultimate determinant of the quality of a product and conformance of the product with specifications as determined through tests and analysis is a fairly accurate and acceptable measure of drug quality. The associations insist that issues such as bioequivalence/bio-availability and stability during shelf life, etc., are raked up to oust the smaller manufacturers from the business.

Manual maintenance and inputting of data and data integrity-related issues have also drawn a lot of criticism. The Indian industry explains these as cultural differences. The experts insist on the uncompromising compliance with best known standards, processes, specifications and data integrity. Many Indian manufacturers also refuse to acknowledge the distinction between therapeutic equivalence and pharmaceutical equivalence of a drug. This has been a subject matter of severe criticism by foreign regulators, other agencies and journalists as drugs that are not therapeutically equivalent fail to produce optimal results when administered to a patient.

Drugs are considered to be therapeutic equivalents only if they are pharmaceutically equivalent and have the same clinical effect and safety profile when administered to patients under conditions specified in the label. They should have been approved as safe and effective; contain identical amounts of the same active drug ingredient in the same dosage form and route of administration; meet the applicable standards of strength, quality, purity and identity; be bioequivalent and manufactured in compliance with the Current Good Manufacturing Practices.[4] Therapeutically equivalent drugs can be used as substitutes of a branded drug. With continuous accretion to the knowledge from the use of medicines over a period of time, the post marketing surveillance, new scientific developments, etc., the quality requirements for medical products continue to undergo upward revision. Therefore, what could have been a quality product a decade back may no longer be considered useful now for any of these reasons.

The Indian pharmaceutical industry has been on the receiving end of the debate on the quality of medical products. There are any numbers of views on the subject – some based on facts, others on hearsay and still others, on pure imagination. No comprehensive and objective study had ever been undertaken to examine the quality of medical products, both from the perspective of the processes followed as well as the product quality, through tests and analysis. Conclusions have continued to be drawn on the basis of small samples, which were, in many cases, as less as ten, subjective

---

[4.] http://bmctoday.net/vehiclesmatter/pdfs/TherapeuticEquivalence.pdf

inputs given by inspectors of different regulators, mostly from the USA and European countries or journalists based on the work of whistle blowers and selected information obtained from regulators. Evidence regarding the deficiencies, including questions about data sufficiency, data reliability and data integrity has been compiled mainly through inspections by regulators of other countries.

In view of the critical role played by medical products in the delivery of health services, it is necessary that there are no compromises with regard to their quality. For this, the regulatory structures should have adequate capacity to exercise quality control. The inadequate capacity of regulators, as brought out in Chapter 2, profit orientation of the industry and corruption has led to therapeutically sub-optimal pharmaceutical products being permitted to be marketed in India and also exported to other countries. In most such cases, the manufactures did not invest enough resources for establishing facilities for testing the stability of drugs over their shelf-life and did not carry out bio-availability/bioequivalence studies with reference to innovator products.

LARGEST EVER DRUG SURVEY: 2014–2016

In the backdrop of stories appearing in the media and elsewhere deprecating the quality of drugs manufactured in India, the MoHFW accorded 'in principle' approval for undertaking a comprehensive survey about the extent of spurious and NSQ drugs in India in the month of April 2014. The task was assigned to the National Institute of Biologicals (NIB), Noida –an autonomous institution of the Government of India. Since a survey of such a magnitude had never been carried out anywhere in the world till then, there was a lot of skepticism and lack of clarity on the issue. In order to ensure that repeated queries did not delay the process, a mechanism was institutionalized to discuss and decide all issues that required government approval.

The NIB was asked to go ahead with the preparatory work without any further delay and focus on ensuring that the survey was conducted in the most professional manner to bring out the true state of affairs. It was also advised that wherever required, the help of the best professional institutions should be availed of for designing the survey or any other activity considered necessary for the smooth conduct of the survey. During the training of personnel associated with the survey work from the government, the non-governmental organizations and the Pharmacy Council of India, the NIB conveyed a loud and clear message that the survey had to be conducted objectively and professionally and no compromise in the process will be tolerated.

When, after following the due process, the private laboratories were being shortlisted for testing and analysis of the samples of the drugs picked up as part of the survey, it turned out that most of the private laboratories that were the lowest bidders were not having the required infrastructure. In a few cases, it was pointed out that some of those laboratories had just one High Performance Liquid Chromatography (HPLC) machine. It was considered that while it would not be appropriate to have the samples tested and analyzed by such laboratories, inviting fresh bids will delay the whole project. However, after detailed discussions, the NIB was asked to go ahead with the design of the survey and other preparatory work.

In order to assess the feasibility of testing the samples within the government laboratories, the Directors of drug testing laboratories were asked to examine the feasibility of testing samples in their facilities. Initially, all Directors indicated that it will not be possible for them to test so many samples and in any case, they neither had the manpower nor the required machinery/equipment for it. They added that given the way the government procurements happen, especially with respect to equipment that had to be imported, it will not be possible to acquire them in time for testing the drugs picked up during the survey.

The Directors of drug testing laboratories were advised that they had an opportunity to strengthen their infrastructure and scale up, and that each laboratory will have to function 24x7. They were assured that the required equipment and additional manpower would be made available to them much before the testing started and refresher courses would be arranged for the staff to ensure that they were familiar with all required processes. A Committee of Directors of laboratories assessed the manpower and equipment requirements and also recommended drug testing laboratories in states that had the required equipment and manpower.

The proposals for procurement of equipment and additional manpower were approved within a week of the receipt of the report of the committee, and orders were placed on M/s HLL for procurement of the approved equipment. Initially, the officials concerned in HLL informed that the procurement will take more than a year. With the intervention of the then Chairman, HLL, the procurement materialized within a record time, and installation and testing of equipment as well as the training of officials was completed before the samples arrived for testing.

Each central drug testing laboratory was also provided additional manpower of 30 to be hired on contractual basis. In addition to training the personnel in the laboratories, specialized training was organized at the Indian Pharmacopoeia Commission, Ghaziabad. Additional samples were collected by the CDSCO field staff for testing in the laboratories so that the staff was fully trained and there were no problems when the survey samples arrived for testing and analysis. The Assistant Drug Inspectors posted at the CDSCO Headquarters were also deputed for training to the Central Drug Testing laboratories for a period of three months. This was done with the twin objective of acquainting them with laboratory work and using their services for drug testing in the event of any contingency.

In the meantime, assured of all necessary approvals, the NIB held detailed discussions with the Indian Statistical Institute, Hyderabad and finalized the drug survey design. Without going into the details of the survey design, etc., it is noteworthy that a sample size of 47,954 drugs was finalized by the NIB and the Indian Statistical Institute, Hyderabad. The survey was unique in many respects and was meticulously planned and executed. It included as many as 15 therapeutic categories and formulations containing 224 drug molecules and selected fixed dose combinations. The samples were picked up from 654 districts and covered retail outlets, government distribution points and the notified ports. To ensure the credibility and transparency of the process, representatives of civil society organizations and the Pharmacy Council of India accompanied all teams deputed for collection of samples. All samples were tested and analyzed in duly certified and accredited drug testing laboratories. The report of the survey is now available in the public domain.[5]

As part of the survey, as many as 69 different tests were performed on samples in laboratories that were specifically equipped and strengthened to ensure strict conformance with test protocols. A total of 47,012 samples were tested. Samples that had expired before being tested and analyzed were excluded. The country-wide survey included drugs from rural areas (25.8%), municipal towns/Taluk Headquarters (46.8%), corporations (22.7%) and metropolitan cities (4.7%).

Based on testing and analysis of the samples collected for the survey, the extent of NSQ and spurious drugs was found to be 3.16% and 0.0245%, respectively, which is more or less at par with what is prevalent in most developed countries. The position with respect to retail outlets was 3% NSQ and 0.023% spurious drugs. It was better than what was prevalent in government supply chain where it was 10.02% and 0.059%, respectively. Within the government sources, NSQ drugs were: civil hospital stores (11.03%), state medical stores (10.44%), ESI dispensaries (9.01%) and CGHS (4.11%).

The quantum of NSQ drugs in the case of 40 manufacturing companies from where 25 or more samples had been drawn was more than the national average of 3%. The highest NSQ drugs were in case of a Gujarat-based company where 90.63% of the samples drawn were found to be NSQ. 11 companies had NSQ drugs in the range of 15% to 90.63% and 27 companies, including some multinational companies, had NSQ drugs exceeding 5%. Some multinational companies had NSQs in excess of 50%.

---

5. http://www.indiaenvironmentportal.org.in/files/file/National%20Drug%20Survey%202014-16.pdf

Surprisingly, of the failed samples, 33.2% failed in the dissolution test, which underpins problems with drug release and its stability and 22.6% samples failed in Assay test, underpinning that the drugs did not contain the required quality of active pharmaceutical ingredient. The findings highlighted serious problems with the government procurement, which largely caters to the poorer strata of the society. In terms of state-wise statistics, Andaman & Nicobar Islands, Puducherry and the North-Eastern states had much higher NSQs. However, the position in large states like Andhra Pradesh, Telangana, Madhya Pradesh, Chhattisgarh, Odisha, Uttar Pradesh, Tamil Nadu, Gujarat, Bihar, etc., was equally bad. The survey findings gave an impression that the manufacturers were not concerned about the quality of the product and were confident that they will be able to manage the regulatory/enforcement structures in the event of any quality compromises being detected.

The drug survey, to a large extent, brought out action points that could improve the quality of medicines in the country.

RISK-BASED INSPECTIONS

The end products when found to be free of contamination and other deficiencies on test and analysis may not necessarily deliver therapeutic benefit promised in the label to the consumer. Further, since many pharmaceutical products had failed during tests and analysis, after analyzing the report of the drug survey conducted during 2014–2016, it was decided that some urgent interventions could help in further addressing the quality, safety and efficacy of medical products in India. This was so as samples of some manufacturers had failed on a very large number of parameters in respect of many products. Further, the failure rate of a few manufacturers was alarmingly high.

In a meeting in the MoHFW, it was noted that there might be something amiss in the processes followed by the manufacturers whose samples had failed repeatedly. It was, therefore, decided that the processes being followed by such manufacturing units particularly with regard to compliance with the Good Manufacturing Practices (GMP)[6] may be reviewed. The review was to include the requirements specified to be fulfilled by the plant and equipment in accordance with the provisions of Schedule 'M' to the Drugs and Cosmetics Rules, 1945 as also international best practices. The WHO GMP and the norms specified by the Pharmaceutical Inspection Convention/ Pharmaceutical Inspection Co-operation (PIC/S) were also taken into account. Accordingly, these were proposed to be included in the detailed check-list prepared for carrying out risk-based inspections.

Knowing that the time was of essence and no time would be more opportune than just after the survey findings to do something to remedy the situation, a team comprising senior officers from the CDSCO, a retired CDSCO Deputy Drug Controller and three retired state drug regulators was constituted to design a detailed tool for conducting risk-based inspections of manufacturing facilities in the country. The methodology for these inspections was also to be used for rating manufacturing sites on the basis of estimated risk that they posed to patients, consumers and animals i.e. the users of medicines, and also take into account the risks to the quality of the product. These modalities were to ensure that the drugs manufactured in the country, at the minimum, complied with the mandatory Good Manufacturing Practices (GMP) and Good Laboratory Practices (GLP) prescribed in the Drugs and Cosmetics Rules, 1945, World Health Organization (WHO) GMP and norms laid down by PIC/S, etc.

With a view to ensuring time-bound action, the team constituted to develop the check-list/toolkit was housed at the NIB, Noida, and all arrangements for their stay, food, transport and other requirements were tied up so that the team could devote itself exclusively to the work assigned to it. The team was asked to prepare the check-list in a very tight schedule for which the reports on NSQ drugs collected from diverse sources, such as the results of the test and analysis undertaken as part of the national

---

6. GMP includes details such as the requirements of premises, surroundings, personnel, sanitation, storage of raw materials, documentation and records, self-inspection and quality control systems and site master files, etc.

survey for determining the quality of drugs in the country; reports of tests and analysis of samples picked up by the central and state regulators; cases where complaints had been received from international regulatory agencies on exported drugs; and other information available with the government, were to be taken into account.

Based on the exercise, the team prepared a comprehensive document for carrying out risk-based inspections. After further discussions, the document was placed in the public domain and information about it was disseminated to all concerned for information, perusal, undertaking self-assessment and taking remedial steps to remove deficiencies without any delay. Industry associations were also advised that inspections will be carried out as per the plan drawn for the purpose and individual manufacturers will be informed of the details before the date of inspection. The toolkit developed for the Risk-based Inspections was later to be adopted for inspecting all pharmaceutical manufacturing units after assessing the efficacy of the toolkit in the first phase.

To ensure the success of the proposed inspections, five one-weeklong training programs were arranged for Assistant Drug Controllers, Drug Inspectors, Assistant Drug Inspectors and Drug Analysts from the central drug testing laboratories. The state governments were also requested to depute drug inspectors and laboratory officials for these training programs. As many as 230 officials from the central and state drug regulatory authorities were trained in five programs organized at the NIB, Noida.

Separately, a core team of officers at the CDSCO Headquarters prepared the lists of manufacturers that were found to be high risk and categorized them into three categories *viz.* those with two or more NSQ drugs; those with three or more NSQ drugs; and those with five or more NSQ drugs during last one year. Keeping in view the repeated complaints about the misuse of oxytocin, its manufacturers were also included in the schedule for inspection. In the first set of inspections, a list of 249 manufacturing sites was finalized for inspection in eight rounds, with each inspection lasting for a period of three days. The inspecting teams were asked to transmit the inspection reports within 48 hours of the inspections having been completed.

These reports were also to be shared with the state licensing authorities and the inspected manufacturing facilities for appropriate corrective action.

OBJECTIONS OF STATE GOVERNMENTS

In accordance with the planned course of action, the selected manufacturing units were informed about the proposed inspection at least a week before the date of inspection. Composite teams headed by an Assistant Drug Controller and comprising drug inspectors from the Centre and the state, and also an analyst from a drug testing laboratory were formed for undertaking inspections. Nomination of inspectors from the state was left to the discretion of the State Licensing Authorities, with the caveat that the drug inspectors and laboratory officials nominated should have undergone training organized for conducting risk-based inspections. It was ensured that no official was deputed for these inspections within the zone in which they were posted.

As soon as copies of the notice for inspection reached manufacturers and state drug regulators, many regulators informed DCG(I) that the proposed inspections were illegal, in excess of the jurisdiction vested in the central government and that the states will not cooperate with the inspecting teams. When this was brought to the notice of MoHFW, DCG(I) was advised to persuade state drug regulators to cooperate in the larger national interest and, in case, they were having difficulty at the governmental level, the issues could be discussed and sorted out.

The DCG(I) and his officers expressed reservations to undertake inspections in the light of serious objections from the state governments. The team was advised that that there was no going back and any lapse in the inspections will be viewed seriously. While most states agreed after discussion with the Additional Chief Secretary/ Principal Secretary concerned, a few states put their foot down. It particularly proved to be a Herculean task to convince the Government of Himachal Pradesh who agreed to the state participating in inspections after detailed discussions on the condition that the modalities of inspection were to be first discussed by the inspecting team with the State Drug Controller. The Tamil Nadu Government also refused to cooperate initially; however, on persuasion, the state government reluctantly agreed.

Many state governments had to be told that the inspections will be undertaken preferably with the states being on board, failing which without states' participation and in the worst-case scenario, irrespective of their objections and non-participation as the CDSCO was legally empowered to do so.

TACTICS TO AVOID INSPECTIONS

The first round of inspections involving 26 manufacturing units was to be carried out in four states *viz.* Tamil Nadu, Maharashtra, Uttarakhand and Himachal Pradesh. Despite assurances over telephone, some of the states did not participate in the inspections and, in some cases, they even created hindrances for the central teams. The ingenuity of some drug manufacturers can be gauged from the fact that while 226 manufacturing units had been included in the schedule for inspections in the first seven rounds and part of the eighth round, actual inspections of only 170 units could take place and 56 identified units could not be inspected.

Out of the units that could not be inspected, production activity was reported to have been stopped in 25 cases, even though the licenses had not been surrendered; manufacturing units were reported to be undergoing renovation in 13 cases; stop production order had been issued by the state drug regulator concerned to one unit; and 10 units had ceased to operate from the approved addresses indicated in the license. In six cases, the licenses had been suspended or cancelled by state licensing authority concerned or the license had expired. In one case, the firm had already been inspected as a loan licensing facility. It was noted that some units in Himachal Pradesh, Uttarakhand and Tamil Nadu were closed temporarily just before the scheduled dates for inspection. It was clear that most of the 56 units did what they did to avoid being subjected to risk-based inspections.

FINDINGS OF THE INSPECTIONS

The inspections revealed that 72% of the manufacturing facilities inspected were not complying with the minimum requirements of schedule 'M' and schedule 'L1' of the Drugs and Cosmetic Rules, 1945, and manufacture of drugs in these units posed a high risk to the stakeholders. The samples of drugs manufactured by these companies had failed consistently. The analysis revealed that out of the first 170 manufacturing plants inspected, the compliance with GMP and GLP in 33 plants was below 25% and importantly, all these plants had many critical deficiencies. 36 of the 170 plants had compliance levels ranging between 25 to 50% and they had deficiencies in critical areas. In case of another 36 plants, the compliance level was between 50 to 75%, with seven of them not having any critical deficiencies. The remaining 65 plants had compliance level higher than 75% and 40 of them had no critical deficiencies. In a case in Tamil Nadu, the inspection team found the premises filthy with open drains while the same company was maintaining a fully WHO GMP compliant facility for manufacturing drugs for exports in the close vicinity of the former.

These inspections brought out that a very large number of drug manufacturing plants were not complying with the prescribed requirements and still they continued to manufacture drugs. The risk-based inspections were carried out in those manufacturing plants where the products had failed repeatedly and to that extent, it is not representative of the entire Indian pharmaceutical industry. Nonetheless, it clearly brings out the chinks in the drug manufacturing process prevalent in the country and underpins the need for urgent reforms, strengthening of processes, improving automation and operating procedures, and religiously following quality management systems in manufacturing plants. It also poses serious questions about the state drug regulators who issue licenses for manufacturing.

STORAGE AND TRANSPORTATION OF DRUGS

Transportation and storage have a profound bearing on the quality of drugs, their efficacy and safety. Drugs of standard quality manufactured after following all necessary protocols when stored or transported in sub-optimal conditions could deteriorate due to the impact of environmental factors such as temperature, air, light and humidity. The shelf-life of drugs is specified keeping, amongst others, the stability of the active pharmaceutical ingredient(s) used in any drug in the ideal storage conditions in view. The stability of drugs is assessed by subjecting them to varying temperature, humidity and other conditions, and observing the impact of such variations on drugs. Drugs lose their efficacy if stored or transmitted in conditions that are not as per specified limits. Improper storage and transmission processes render the drugs unfit for human and animal use.

Drugs that have been transported or stored in conditions different from the prescribed ones may not remain fit for human or animal use. Their use could harm the patient and also pose greater risk in terms of antimicrobial resistance. Proper storage and transmission of drugs is, as such, a key requirement for ensuring their quality, safety and efficacy. To that extent, transportation and storage of drugs is a highly specialized job, and appropriately qualified and sensitized manpower has to be deployed for handling these aspects.

Depending on the climatic conditions, drugs are generally required to be stored in dry, well-ventilated premises at temperatures ranging between 15 and 25°C. In some cases, storage could be permitted up to a maximum temperature of 30°C. Separate storage conditions are specified for special products like vaccines, etc. In keeping with the stability requirements of the product, the recommended storage conditions are required to be prominently indicated on the label of the drug and meticulously followed for retaining their quality and efficacy.

The storage requirements for medicines in India are specified in the Drugs and Cosmetics Rules, 1945 – a subordinate legislation framed under the Drugs and Cosmetics Act, 1940. As per these rules, it is the primary responsibility of those engaged in storage and distribution of medicines to take steps to ensure that the quality of medicines and integrity of distribution chain is maintained throughout the distribution process – from the site of the manufacturer till dispensing to the patient.

Materials and pharmaceutical products need to be handled and stored carefully to prevent contamination, mix-ups and cross-contamination. The areas selected for storage of medicines should be neat, clean, dry and free from accumulated waste and vermin. Depending upon the products stored, the temperature of storage areas has to be maintained within *the* prescribed limits. The storage area has to be large enough to allow orderly storage of different products and also be well-lit so that necessary activities could be undertaken accurately and safely. In case of products requiring special storage, conditions indicated on the label such as range of temperature, relative humidity, etc., are required to be followed and conformance with such conditions needs to be ensured, checked, monitored and recorded meticulously.

Materials and pharmaceutical products are not to be stored on the floor and adequate space has to be left for cleaning the area and for undertaking inspection. Pallets need to be kept in a good state of cleanliness and repair. A written sanitation document indicating the frequency of cleaning and the methods to be used for cleaning the premises and storage areas is required to be prepared, maintained and displayed prominently. Similarly, a written document specifying the measures required to be taken for pest control along with details of safe agents that can be used to obviate any risk of contamination of materials and pharmaceutical products has to be maintained.

Appropriate procedures for cleaning any spillage to ensure removal of a possible risk of contamination are required to be kept handy, and care has to be taken to ensure that the staff is fully aware of these procedures. Highly active and radioactive materials, narcotics and other hazardous, sensitive and/or dangerous materials and pharmaceutical products, as well as substances presenting special risks of abuse, fire or explosion, are required to be stored in a dedicated area with appropriate additional safety and security measures.

One of the essential requirements concerning storage of medicines is that the records should be maintained properly. Any compromise in record keeping could be construed as tampering with *the* documents and raise doubts about data integrity. Equipment used for monitoring need to be checked at suitable pre-determined intervals, and results of such checking recorded and retained for the duration of the shelf-life of the stored material or product plus one year. Temperature monitors should ideally be located in areas that are most likely to show fluctuations and temperature mapping should show uniformity of temperature throughout the storage facility.

INSPECTION OF BULK STORAGE FACILITIES

Keeping in view the impact of transportation and storage on the quality of drugs, surprise inspections of bulk storage facilities across the country were planned in March 2017. The step was considered necessary for maintaining the quality, safety and efficacy of medical products marketed in the country through compliance with prescribed norms for transportation and storage of drugs as part of the efforts to cleanse the system. The first surprise inspection was scheduled to be carried out in Bhagirath Palace,[7] Delhi on June 9, 2017.

Bhagirath Palace, a dusty, tightly packed market in Chandni Chowk, Old Delhi, houses wholesale licensed drug distributors, Delhi's key wholesale electrical and lights, and medical appliances markets. The markets have no fire extinguishers and electrical and telephone wires are out in the open. It would appear to be the most unsuitable place for storage of large quantities of medical products. A fire had broken out in the electrical market in Bhagirath Palace on December 13, 2012 and the authorities could not control the fire for days as entering the narrow lanes was nearly impossible.

[7.] Bhagirath Palace has an interesting history of its own and a peep into that, despite not being relevant for the present work, would be in order. This 18th century Old Delhi Palace, presently known as Bhagirath Palace, was once the *haveli* (palace) of a Kashmiri nautch girl, Begum Samru, who led a band of mercenaries and was a close aid of Mughal emperors. Begum Samru later rose to be the ruler of Sardhana in Meerut. The palace was a symbol of power and sex two centuries ago. It was privy to many conspiracies and mechanizations concerning royalty and whispers between lovers. Till India's independence, the palace continued to be known as Begum Samru's Palace. After independence, it was bought by LalaBhagirath Mal. The 200-year-old structure, now lying in a dilapidated state, echoes with the cacophony of hawkers and witnesses heavy traffic during business hours.

The licensed drug distributors, around 400 in numbers, operate from multiple buildings such as Jagsonpal building, Central Bank of India Building, etc., in Bhagirath Palace. Business worth thousands of crore of rupees is transacted from this place every year and it serves as the nodal point for supplying medicines to most states in north India. Due to paucity of storage space, most of the shops have built attics of around 3 feet height, accessible only through narrow stairways or even temporary ladders from inside the licensed premises. In many cases, access to upper floors and basement areas has also been provided from within the licensed premises. Buildings in the market are not equipped with any fire extinguishers to deal with any unfortunate mishap. Even without going into the findings of inspection, any layman would come to the conclusion that keeping in view the dilapidated condition of the infrastructure, the place could not have been permitted to have so many establishments, including those storing life-saving medical products.

Initially, selected officials were deployed in the area to familiarize themselves with the location, topography and observe activities and gather information. A team of four drugs inspectors was constituted who gathered information and visited Bhagirath Palace *in cognito* several times and identified shops where large-scale contraventions were taking place. The team reported on a daily basis to the Joint Drug Controller, who kept the DCG(I) informed of the developments.

A total of 142 officials of the CDSCO were identified for carrying out surprise inspection and were divided into 27 teams. On June 8, 2017, the selected officials were imparted detailed instructions on how the inspections were to be carried out and what precautions were to be taken. However, where and at what time the inspections were to be conducted was kept a secret till the actual operations on June 9, 2017.

At 9:30 AM of June 9, 2017, Police Commissioner, Delhi was requested to deploy police to assist the CDSCO team. The DCG(I) personally briefed the Delhi Police Commissioner on the issue. A police team of 50 led by a Deputy Commissioner of Police provided protection to the inspecting teams. The inspections started at around 12.30 PM as activity in the market picks up only around noon. Just a few minutes before commencing inspections, Delhi Drugs Control Department officials were also requested to participate in the inspection.

As soon as the news of *the* surprise inspections reached shopkeepers, many shops were shut down by the owners. The CDSCO officials could inspect only 57 licensed wholesalers, including warehouses. The exercise revealed shocking transgressions that had the potential to jeopardize human life and certainly compromise healthcare. What was most worrisome was the fact that all such transgressions were happening in the capital city under the nose of the central government and at a distance of five kilometers from the headquarters of the CDSCO.

The inspection revealed that the available space in all establishments was much below the prescribed requirements and the quantum of medicines stored was many times more than the capacity of those shops. A majority of the licensed premises were having an area of less than 10 square meters stipulated as the minimum requirement under the Drugs & Cosmetics Rules, 1945 for such establishments, resulting in congestion and poor storage conditions. The storage space for drugs and working space for personnel was found to be inadequate and attics of 3 feet height were being used by most of the wholesalers. The attic space had no ventilation, fire protection, cold storage facilities or even proper working space for a person. Consignments of drugs awaiting shipment to customers were stored in open corridors and also on streets as there was no space in the licensed premises and warehouses.

The inspection also revealed that drugs labeled as 'Store in cool place' (8–25 degrees centigrade) were stored at room temperature (at around 40 degrees centigrade) during the hot and humid summer of Delhi. Finished Formulations, including those of antibiotic, antibacterial, antihypertensive, cardiovascular, oncology, anti-diabetic drugs labeled as 'Store in a cool place', were haphazardly dumped in warehouses without having any cold storage facilities and without space for entry and exit of personnel. In a number of cases, the refrigerators meant for storage of drugs requiring

2–8 degrees centigrade were either switched off or used for refrigeration of food, water and beverages.

It was revealed that vaccines such as Tetanus Toxoid requiring storage at 2–8 degrees centigrade were either stocked in thermo-coal boxes containing ice packs or kept on open racks and shelves. The manpower handling stored products used packed shippers containing medicines as ladders to fetch goods from the attic. In most cases, the staff walked from one part of the shop to another on boxes of medicines. Drugs were being handled by workmen who were not qualified or trained for the job. They were completely ignorant about the processes involved in handling and storage of medicines.

It was noted that corrugated boxes containing drugs had been stacked on each other and the tertiary packing of products was being done on the streets, in open air and directly on the floor. The overall hygiene in the shops and surrounding areas was abysmal, with stinking washrooms and debris littered all around. The inspection revealed that accidental exposure to cytotoxic drugs on account of spillages and breakage could not be ruled out due to poor storage and distribution practices. The inspection also brought out that the competent persons were not aware of the consequences of such accidents and procedures to be followed in such cases.

The personnel engaged were also not aware of storage conditions for vaccines, thermo-labile products, etc. Purchase and distribution records of products were not maintained and stock ledgers were not updated regularly. Relevant persons were also not aware of the safe disposal practices required to be followed for expired drugs and methods to be followed for return of drugs to manufacturers in the event of any drug safety alert or drug recall.

It also revealed a lot of inconsistencies in documentation. In 17 instances, the wholesale dealers were not able to produce purchase bills. In one instance, the person carrying the goods ran away, leaving the goods on the road when questioned about the source of drugs. The quantities purchased, sold and the stock remaining after sale did not tally in almost all cases. Lack of traceability as to from where the drugs had been purchased posed a serious question mark on the genuineness of the supply chain, and the possibility of introduction of spurious products in the supply chain could not be ruled out. Drugs were distributed to retailers without delivery note or invoices and transactions were mostly based on telephonic orders. The name and address of the consignee and consignor for the drugs in transit remained unclear. Copies of electronically generated and signed sale invoices were not maintained for verification, and electronic stock distribution records were operated and maintained by the staff other than the competent persons. The list of drugs and their location in the warehouse had not been documented and bin card system or records of purchase and distribution to reflect the quantity in hand in warehouses was not maintained.

It was also noted that all establishments in the area relied on power supply from the state power utilities for operation of refrigerators and deep freezers for storage of medicines, including oncology products and vaccines. However, no arrangements had been made for power backup in any of the establishments that could be inspected by the team. In brief, the wholesale dealers were found not to be complying with most of the prescribed storage conditions. It was noted that licenses had been issued to them in complete disregard to the provisions of law.

It could be anybody's guess if the state of affairs in other wholesale locations was any different. Whatever the inspection revealed, speaks very poorly of the storage and distribution practices in vogue and it poses a serious threat to millions of unsuspecting consumers. If this could happen in the capital city that also houses the national regulator, the position in far-flung areas can only be imagined.

OTHER GROUND REALITIES

It has been noticed that the facilities that manufactured medicines for export to highly regulated markets were compliant with the best international practices and all possible precautions had been taken in accordance with the requirements of Indian GMP, WHO GMP as well as the specific requirements stipulated by regulators of importing countries, particularly the USFDA. It would be rather difficult, in most such cases, to find fault with those facilities. Companies manufacturing for export to the developed world were found to be making a conscious effort to comply with the strictest quality control norms. However, with ever increasing regulatory rigors of importing countries, even these manufacturers sometimes failed to meet the required standards as quality requirements continue to be scaled up. The facilities for manufacturing products for export to well-regulated markets are world class and are substantially superior to the ones manufacturing medicines for the Indian market and export to lesser regulated markets.

It is important to take note of the fact that those who adhere to quality standards cannot compete in terms of prices with what is referred to as 'Kadhai Chhap'[8] manufacturers, some of whom were, at one time, traders and had little expertise in manufacturing quality medicines. Consequently, in most cases under the L-I criteria used in government procurements, the latter succeed in tenders to supply medicines to government health facilities. A major reason for the dual standards is the proliferation of the fly-by-night operators due to lax regulation in the country and exploitation of loopholes for profiteering at the cost of public health and public good. The lax regulation allows Even the non-licensed facilities continue to manufacture drugs, medical devices and cosmetics. The higher percentage of NSQ drugs in government supply chain is directly relatable to this.

The concerns expressed at different forums regarding spurious, adulterated and NSQ drugs manufactured and marketed in the country and exported to other markets that do not have stringent regulations for medical products are all in the possession of the government and the CDSCO. The diplomatic officials of various countries had, during the course of their meetings in the MoHFW, also raised concerns in this regard. Besides the findings of the USFDA and other regulators, the papers available in the Ministry include complaints received from countries such

---

8. *Kadhai* is a utensil used for preparing vegetables in Indian kitchens. The term 'Kadhai Chhap' refers to the very rudimentary style of doing something.

as Sri Lanka, Vietnam, Russia, Ghana, amongst others, about the quality of drugs sourced from India.

In most complaints received by the Ministry, the state governments concerned informed that the medicines had, in those cases, been supplied through trade channels rather than having been sourced directly from the manufacturers. The manufacturers of the NSQ drugs could not be traced in majority of the cases of such complaints. In a few cases, it was noticed that there were no licensed manufacturers conforming to the names, addresses or descriptions printed on the labels of medicines.

It is apparent that the end-products of those manufacturers who do not adhere to required processes during manufacturing also fail more often on test and analysis, and there are a large number of them. In India, the quality of the medical products is affected not only because of the problems with the manufacturing processes and the quality of raw materials or API/KSM/DI but also due to the improper storage and transportation of such products. The findings of drug survey, risk-based inspections, inspection of wholesale drug storage facilities and prevalence of drugs manufactured by unknown entities highlight that all is not well with the so-called pharmacy of the world.

Quality is an essential and basic requirement and cannot be confined to the end products meeting specified parameters; it also needs to take into account the way each manufacturing unit and sub-units follow the prescribed work processes to manufacture, transport, store and dispense medical products. The three aspects discussed in this chapter clearly spell out the actionable points that should be addressed without any delay.

CHAPTER 5

AVARICIOUSNESS, CONNIVANCE AND CORRUPTION

BUSINESS IS MORE THAN JUST MAKING MONEY

Money is central to any business. Doing business is, however, not just about minting more money or profits. Successful businessmen create new products and services that positively impact the lives of people. Successful businessmen know for sure that investing in new innovations or engaging in creativity for enhancing customer experience holds the key to building a sustainable and profitable enterprise. They, therefore, take all possible steps to enhance the experience of existing customers, onboard new customers and win their trust and support. The spin-off of such a customer-centric approach is more wealth in the hands of enterprising businessmen and also increased consumer satisfaction.

In many cases, the business is accompanied by gluttony, which reduces the businessmen to a ravenous jungle beast intensely focused on minting money through means, fair or foul. A corporate which is even tacitly permissive of greed, encourages unethical behavior, starts equating profit with greed, and that is the beginning of the slide down. In an organization that condones or permits disreputable demeanor, the ethical conduct –both at the corporate and individual levels –gets displaced by an insatiable greed. Making profit at all costs becomes the sole objective and the guiding philosophy of the organization. Greed is bottomless, just like the barren desert that sucks in all rain but still does not support life. It has a self-propelling mechanism with no brakes and no limits. The avariciousnesss often concomitant of corruption sets in motion a chain of events that propels and leads to the eventual decline and fall of the enterprise and at a huge cost to the customers and the society. Very often, such a decline is not confined to a single enterprise and could engulf the entire industry unless remedial measures are activated on time. There can be no disaster greater than such covetousness being aided, facilitated and abetted by the structures that are supposed to be guarding against it, especially in a noble field such as human health.

The chapter briefly recapitulates how the Fixed Dose Combinations (FDCs), a highly useful innovation in the field of medical science, were misused for minting profits without caring for human health. The greed of a few businessmen, the inactions and omissions of regulators, bureaucrats and political executive in permitting and perpetuating the continued marketing of irrational FDCs in India represents an unholy and lethal alliance. The entire story of irrational FDCs illustrates how the corporate greed leads to the degeneration of the moral fabric of an entire industry and governmental structures without being mindful of the wrong it has perpetuated. One comes to the irresistible conclusion that the irrational FDCs continue to be marketed in India with the tacit aid, understanding and even encouragement of authorities concerned. The Indian judiciary has also contributed in the process.

Before 2014, the central regulator and the central government did make some feeble efforts before 2014, including issuing directions to state regulators. But soft pedaling could not stop the perpetuation of unapproved FDCs, rational and irrational. It was only in 2014 that the decisive steps taken under the directions of the then Minister of Health and Family Welfare, including expeditious examination by a committee headed by an eminent academician, set the course for prohibition of 349 irrational FDCs, only to be frustrated through judicial processes. All this, however, did not help the cause of health as FDCs that have no therapeutic justification continued to be marketed. The chapter also raises a serious question about the limits of such intervention by the judiciary, particularly on procedural grounds in matters concerning science.

FIXED DOSE COMBINATIONS AND THEIR RATIONALITY

A combination of two or more drugs combined in a fixed ratio is called a Fixed Dose Combination (FDC). Very often, the treatment protocol requires administering more than one medicine for treatment of certain conditions. FDCs in which more than one medicine have been combined is an innovation that makes the treatment process simpler and helps in overcoming difficulties associated in administering multiple medicines to a patient. Broadly, when two or more drugs are combined, the emerging combination is altogether a new drug. The impact of combining drugs could have one of the three possible effects *viz.* (i) the new drug could, as a result of synergy, have increased potency or simply put, result in value addition; (ii) the potency of the new combination may remain unaltered, i.e., equivalent to the total of the potency of two drugs taken separately or a situation of no value addition; and (iii) reduced potency of the new combination as a result of the ingredients of the FDC counteracting each other and reducing the utility of either one or both ingredients.

Based on the above, the FDCs can be classified as the Good ones, having strong justification; the Bad ones, formulated primarily with marketing interests and with no value addition in terms of therapeutic usefulness and whose justification is debatable; and the Ugly ones that have neither evidence nor theoretical justifications of any value addition and on the contrary, result in reduced benefit to the consumer.

An article in the *Indian Journal of Pharmacology* listed the benefits of FDCs.[1] The authors have propositioned that the FDCs are justified when they demonstrate clear benefits in terms of (a) potentiating therapeutic efficacy; (b) reducing the incidence of adverse effect of drugs; (c) having pharmacokinetic[2] advantage; (d) better compliance by reducing the pill burden; (e) reduced dose of individual drugs; (f) lower resistance to the drug; and (g) reduction in the cost of medication as compared with an individual drug due to cost of packaging, distribution, etc. In short, such FDCs improve the utility of the innovation to the consumer. However, all

---

[1.] Yogendra Kumar Gupta and Suganthi S. RamachandranIndian J Pharmacology 2016 Jul–Aug; 48(4): 347–349. doi: 10.4103/0253-7613.186200PMCID: PMC4980918 PMID: 27756941 Fixed dose drug combinations: Issues and challenges in India.

[2.] Pharmacokinetics refers to a study of the bodily absorption, distribution, metabolism and excretion of drugs or the characteristic interactions of a drug and the body in terms of its absorption, distribution, metabolism and excretion

innovations are not necessarily inspired by public good. There could be some that are influenced purely by greed and while not making any value addition, could even be harmful to patients.

The authors have in the above referred article added that the FDCs formulated without due diligence can pose multiple problems including: (a) pharmacodynamic[3] mismatch between two components, one drug having additive/antagonistic effect, leading to reduced efficacy or enhanced toxicity; (b) pharmacokinetic mismatch and having peak efficacy at different lengths of time; (c) chemical non-compatibility leading to decreased shelf life; (d) drug interactions because of the common metabolizing pathways; and (e) limitations of finer dosing titration[4] of individual ingredients.

Many FDCs being marketed in India combine drugs that have the opposite impact. For example, professionals in the field inform that most of the cough-cold remedies in the Indian market were a combination of an expectorant and a suppressant. In the process of treatment of cough and cold, the options are either to remove the phlegm in the respiratory system by using an expectorant or in case of an irritating cough with no or insignificant amount of phlegm, to suppress it. Both removal and suppression of phlegm cannot be achieved at the same time. Any combination of an expectorant and a suppressant will, therefore, only confuse the body mechanism and worsen the condition of the patient. Such FDCs are clearly irrational and there can be no logic other than pure greed to justify why such irrational FDCs should have been introduced in the first place.

Another important aspect that needs to be taken into account is the half-life of the drugs combined in the FDCs. The elimination of half-life of a drug is a pharmacokinetic parameter and represents the time taken for the concentration of the drug in the plasma or the amount of the drug in the body to be reduced by 50%. With ingredients combined in an FDC

[3.] Pharmacodynamic is the study of the relationship between the concentration of a drug at the site of action and its biochemical and physiological effect.

[4.] A titration is a technique where a solution of known concentration is used to determine the concentration of an unknown solution.

with half-lives of different durations, it will be impossible to prescribe an optimal dose of such a cocktail as one of the two drugs will remain in the body for a longer duration. In India, half-life of the molecules included in many FDCs has a difference of many hours. Apparently, FDCs containing drugs with different half-lives are irrational and do not enhance consumer welfare. The only consequence of such an irrational combination would either be an overdose of the drug with higher half-life leading to increased toxicity that could have fatal consequences in some cases or under-dose of the drug with lower half-life, opening up the possibility of antimicrobial resistance in FDCs containing antibiotics. In either case, it would be harmful not only to the patient under treatment but also pose a serious challenge to the utility of otherwise efficacious antibiotics in future.

MANUFACTURE OF UNAPPROVED FDCS

In term of the Drugs and Cosmetics Rules, 1945, as they were after amendment to these rules in 1980s, the FDCs combined for the first time were included under the definition of a new drug, and before issuing licenses for their manufacture, approval of the CDSCO was necessary. The CDSCO was, in terms of these rules, *inter alia*, responsible for handling matters relating to product approval, approval of standards, clinical trials, introduction of new drugs and import licenses for new drugs. An FDC being a new drug could, as such, have been licensed for manufacturing in a state only if it had been approved by the CDSCO after examining the data on rationality, safety and efficacy of the proposed combination.

The FDCs were conceived with the noble objective of improving healthcare outcomes. The goal of the innovation was primarily to reduce the burden of the patients and the psychological impact of taking too many pills, or put in simpler words – to enhance consumer satisfaction. Unfortunately, in pursuance of the philosophy of 'greed is good 'in case of the Indian pharmaceutical industry, the avariciousness accompanied by risky unprofessional behavior flirting with illegality has acquired epidemic proportions. The manufacturing of irrational FDCs which sought to bypass the price controls put in place by the National Pharmaceutical Pricing Authority (NPPA), demonstrates the naked dance by arrogant manufacturers, facilitated by state authorities concerned.

To keep the reader fully on board, it is clarified that all medicines included in the National List of Essential Medicines (NLEM) in India are invariably subject to price control by NPPA. The new FDCs that come into being after the NLEM had been finalized would normally not be under the price control mechanism till the revision of the NLEM some years later. The manufacturers would, in such a situation, be free to charge higher prices for such FDCs, if permitted to be manufactured.

Spruced by cupidity which possibly found its grand natural ally in corruption, a lot many manufacturers joined the FDC bandwagon mainly with the purpose of minting profits by browbeating price controls. The mad rush for newer FDCs in India became a universal obsession for drug manufacturers. The state licensing authorities, despite repeated directives from the CDSCO and the MoHFW to stop issuing such licenses, continued to issue licenses for manufacturing and marketing FDCs without their safety, efficacy and quality having been assessed. As a result, the Indian market was flooded with the largest number of FDCs in the world, which includes the ones that are outright irrational and do not have any therapeutic utility.

Initially, as the Indian pharmaceutical industry was still developing and the regulatory structures were largely non-existent or existed only for namesake, knowledge about the harmful effects of such FDCs was inadequate. At the same time, the number of FDCs being manufactured was insignificant. However, with the accumulation of new scientific knowledge and improved regulatory practices followed elsewhere, the possible damage from such FDCs became clearer and that led to changes in the relevant rules mandating approval of the CDSCO for introduction of new FDCs.

Most of the Indian pharmaceutical companies manufacturing FDCs not approved by the CDSCO were aware that their action to obtain licenses for manufacturing FDCs from the state regulators was illegal and unethical. They were also cognizant of the fact that the approval from the CDSCO will be a time-consuming process, and the approval might not come through in many cases due to the proposed combinations not being rational. Of course, it would not be out of place to mention that the CDSCO would also not have been fully equipped for handling so many applications and it did not have the necessary in-house expertise and capacity to handle such a huge influx.

The manufacturers invented shortcuts to mint quick profit and it did not matter whether such actions were contrary to law and might give rise to public health concerns. Actions of the state drug regulators who illegally permitted such combinations to be manufactured and the drug manufacturers who sought such approvals and manufactured FDCs, posed serious risk to human health and life. In a way, they were partners in subverting the law and their actions would have, in normal course, entailed deterrent punishment not only for violation of the Drugs & Cosmetics Act and Rules but also for posing serious risk to public health. However, the state drug regulators and the drug manufacturers not only flouted the law with impunity but also sought to justify their actions and obtain *post facto* legal sanction for such illegal activities. In the face of such arrogance of both the state regulators and the manufacturers, the response of the central government has largely been limited to issuance of circulars and advisories. In any case, in matters that could affect human health, it is inconceivable that an illegal action could be ratified *post facto* and made legal.

LOBBYING BY MANUFACTURERS

Despite sharp differences on a number of issues, all associations of drug manufacturers in India have been *ad idem* on regularization of unapproved FDCs manufactured illegally. These associations as well as individual manufacturers have lobbied for regularization of FDCs at political as well as at bureaucratic levels.

The lobbying for regularization of FDCs used to intensify every time there was a change in senior management position. In July and August 2014, the associations of drug manufacturers made presentations in the

MoHFW highlighting, *inter alia*, that the FDCs had been in use for so long without any problem and should, therefore, be allowed to be marketed. The two main arguments mustered by them to justify the demand were: (a) when two drugs administered individually are not harmful, how could the combination thereof be harmful? and (b) the then DCG(I) had reportedly in one of the meetings with the manufacturers' associations in Baddi, Himachal Pradesh assured that the exercise of calling for applications was a mere formality and the FDCs will be approved after necessary fee had been paid and paper work completed.

DIRECTIONS TO WITHDRAW 294 FDCS

The first major attempt to initiate corrective action and restore some semblance of order was made in 2007, when the CDSCO prepared a list of 294 unapproved FDCs and issued directions to withdraw them from the market under Section 33P of the Drugs & Cosmetics Act, 1940.This was, however, a half-hearted effort and lacked ownership. In hindsight, after perusal of the facts of the case, one would wonder whether it was at all meant to be pursued to a logical conclusion or was it an exercise taken up only for name's sake.

On the pleas of pharmaceutical manufacturers, the Madras High Court had granted a stay that continued till the matter was disposed of by the Supreme Court in December 2017, after the case was, on an application of the MoHFW, transferred to the Supreme Court from the Madras High Court. In the process, the irrational FDCs that had been adjudged to be unsafe from the angles of quality, safety and efficacy or therapeutic considerations, continued to be marketed for more than a decade! From the pace of the proceedings in the matter in the Madras High Court, it appeared that the fact that marketing of such FDCs could jeopardize the lives of millions did not bother the system.

The problem of irrational FDCs was, however, not restricted to these 294 FDCs, and some state regulators were still going ahead full steam and issuing licenses for manufacturing FDCs. On two occasions, the DCG(I) deputed his officers to meet the state regulators and advise them to cancel the licenses issued by them. The issue was also repeatedly flagged in the meetings of the Drug Consultative Committee, and state regulators were advised to desist from issuing licenses for manufacturing unapproved FDCs. A few state regulators mentioned that they were under pressure from state governments as the industry had started relocating to places where licenses for manufacturing unapproved FDCs were issued without any difficulty.

EXAMINATION BY PARLIAMENTARY STANDING COMMITTEE

The Parliamentary Standing Committee on Health and Family Welfare had, in its 59th Report given in May 2012,[5] flagged the issue regarding flooding of the Indian market with many FDCs that had not been assessed for efficacy or safety or approved by the CDSCO. The Committee noted that in these cases, the state licensing authorities had issued manufacturing licenses contrary to the provisions of the Drugs & Cosmetics Rules, 1945. The Standing Committee had also pointed out that such FDCs posed a significant risk to human beings and needed to be withdrawn immediately from the market. The Standing Committee had asked the government to frame a clear and transparent policy for approving FDCs based on scientific principles. It suggested that Section 26A of the Drugs & Cosmetic Act be used to deal with the problem of FDCs not approved by the CDSCO.[6]

[5.] Available at: http://164.100.47.5/newcommittee/reports/EnglishCommittees/Committee%20on%20 Health%20 and%20 Family%20Welfare/59.pdf

[6.] Section 26A of the Drugs & Cosmetics Act, 1940 empowers the Central Government to regulate, restrict or prohibit the manufacture, sale or distribution of a drug or a cosmetic in public interest if it is satisfied that the use of any drug or cosmetic is likely to involve any risk to human beings or animals or that any drug does not have the therapeutic value claimed or purported to be claimed for it or contains ingredients and in such quantity for which there is no therapeutic justification and in the public interest, it is necessary or expedient to do so.

THE ART OF NOT TAKING DECISIONS

Decision making, especially in complex cases, is a difficult skill, even in smaller organizations. It is much more difficult in governmental structures where both external and internal factors, including political considerations, economic uncertainties, legal consequences, inhospitable organizational structures, inept leadership or de-motivated human resources, impact the process. In such circumstances, a seasoned public administrator invariably looks for a way out for deferring the decision, knowing well that his tenure in the organization is limited and it will pass. They know the advantages of not taking the bull by its horns and also understand the unpleasant nuances of having to face the Central Bureau of Investigation, the Central Vigilance Commission or attract the indictment of the Comptroller & Auditor General of India.

A very useful and oft-practiced trick in such situations is to refer the matter to a committee or a group of officers or experts. It would provide them sufficient leeway. The current generation of Indian administrators is cognizant of the fact that the responsibility is generally fixed for taking decisions, especially when they go wrong, and there is invariably no accountability for not taking decisions. There are any number of examples of bureaucrats who rose to the highest positions in the government and did not work long enough in any organization to be held accountable for anything because during their short tenures in different organizations, they made no decisions.

An Additional Secretary in the Ministry of Defence as early as 1986 fondly narrated an anecdote that the Chief Secretary of his home cadre only wrote two words on files throughout his career with the government. When the file was put up, he wrote, 'submitted'; and when it was to go down, he wrote, 'immediate', and he rose to be the Chief Secretary of the state! Perils of decision making on the other hand are manifested by those who had to face conviction and even imprisonment post retirement, in many cases, for taking decisions that could, without the benefit of hindsight, be considered fully in sync with the stated government policy and also in the larger public interest.

The handling of the matter concerning FDCs by the government amply demonstrates the perfection achieved in not making decisions. In the light of the report of the Standing Committee of Parliament on the subject, instead of withdrawing the unapproved FDCs from the market, the government, in October 2012, issued directions to states and union territories under Section 33P of the Drugs & Cosmetics Act, 1940 not to grant licenses for manufacturing FDCs falling under the definition of 'new drugs' that had not been approved by the CDSCO.

The fact that instead of acting on the advice of the Standing Committee of Parliament to invoke Section 26A of the Drugs & Cosmetics Act, 1940, the government decided to invite applications from the manufacturers of FDCs for possible *post facto* regularization of the illegally manufactured drugs manifests the clout the pharmaceutical industry wields. The DCG(I) requested all state drug controllers to ask the manufacturers concerned in their respective states/union territories to prove the safety and efficacy of FDCs within a period of 18 months where licenses for manufacture had been issued prior to 01.10.2012 without approval of the CDSCO. It was added that in the event of the failure to prove safety and efficacy, the manufacturing and marketing of FDCs will be considered for being prohibited in the country. On 05.07.2013, the DCG(I) advised state drug controllers to ask manufacturers to apply, as per the procedure prescribed, within the 18-month period to the CDSCO for regularization or otherwise of FDCs licensed by state regulators without CDSCO's approval. The CDSCO received over 6300 applications in accordance with this advisory.

While opinions are bound to differ, it is considered that the decision taken by the government in the aftermath of severe indictment by the Standing Committee of Parliament was not correct. It cannot be anybody's case that I shall contravene the law and, thereafter, seek approval for legitimizing the wrong. *Prima facie,* anything not manufactured legally in the first place should have been forced to be withdrawn from the market or prohibited, and criminal proceedings initiated against drug manufacturers and the state drug regulators held responsible for issuing licenses for manufacturing something outside their competence and jurisdiction. A polity governed by the rule of law cannot permit such deliberate violation of the law, especially when actions of manufacturers and the state regulators posed a serious threat to millions of users across the globe and clearly violated the law of the land.

EXAMINATION OF ISSUES BY COMMITTEES

Be that as it may be, the CDSCO managed a way out. With the approval of the Ministry, it constituted 10 Expert Committees for examining applications received by it for regularization of FDCs. However, since the said Committees could examine only about 295 applications up to September 2014, the then Minister of Health and Family Welfare, Dr. Harsh Vardhan, directed constitution of a Committee under the Chairmanship of Professor C.K. Kokate, Vice Chancellor, KLE University, Belgaum, Karnataka for examining their safety and efficacy. The orders constituting Kokate Committee were issued on September 16, 2014. It must be stated that this step of Dr. Harsh Vardhan was perhaps the first action in the right direction in the given circumstances. The fact that he was a politician cast in a different mold and also a practicing professional who knew the gravity of the problem, enabled a quick decision in the matter.

Dr. Vardhan was later shifted to the Ministry of Science & Technology. Credit must also be given to his successor, JP Nadda, who neither interfered in the process of examination by the Kokate committee nor even spoke to any officials on the issue, and allowed the process to be completed in a transparent and scientific manner. This was despite the fact that the drug manufacturers from his home state of Himachal Pradesh had been pressing hard to permit continuation of the FDCs.

As advised by the MoHFW, the Kokate Committee organized additional meetings on Saturdays, Sundays and other holidays. The progress was reviewed on a weekly basis in the Ministry. In the meantime, somehow, the then Secretary, Health and Family Welfare got the impression that the CDSCO was delaying the process of finalization of the report. While the file was put up to him to apprise him of the progress of the examination of the matter by the committee, he noted that the progress was slow, and he stated that he will be forced to take action against the officials concerned if the report is delayed. Since the matter was being monitored tightly and regularly, the file was sent back to the then Secretary, pointing out that the impression gained by him was erroneous and the committee's work was progressing at a reasonably good pace. Later, the DCGI was advised that the pace be further hastened and if required, additional manpower be positioned at the disposal of the committee to gather information and assist it.

The Kokate Committee categorized the applications received from the manufacturers of FDCs in four categories *viz.* (a) 963 Irrational FDCs; (b) 1738 FDCs requiring further deliberation; (c) 2617 Rational FDCs; and (d) 309 FDCs requiring Phase IV trials, and submitted the First assessment report to the government on 19.01.2015.The report was approved by the Ministry on 08.05.2015. After acceptance of the report, the CDSCO issued 'Show cause notices' to all manufacturers of FDCs assessed as irrational and also issued approval letters in respect of rational FDCs to the applicants. In case of irrational FDCs, replies to the show cause notices were placed for examination before the Kokate Committee.

In order to ensure an objective assessment and also that injustice was not done to anyone, the committee was assisted by the best subject matter experts drawn from the top-most medical institutions of the country. The Committee submitted its final report to the Ministry on 10.02.2016. Thereafter, in order to assess the report, presentations were made by the Committee before the Secretary, MoHFW, in which it was decided that the reasons for the recommendations with respect to each FDC may be added to the report.

PROHIBITION OF 344 FDCS

The Kokate Committee report was examined in the Ministry and put up for approval of the Minister of Health and Family Welfare and based on examination, 344 notifications were published in the *Gazette of India* on March 10, 2016, prohibiting 344 FDCs. Subsequently, the government prohibited five more FDCs on 08.06.2017 after examination of the observations of the Parliamentary Standing Committee contained in its 59th report and subsequent consultation with the New Drugs Advisory Committee.

In a pre-scheduled meeting in the MoHFW on 14.03.2016, a delegation of the representatives of the Indian Pharmaceutical Alliance enquired whether there was any proposal to ban FDCs. The delegation was informed that the notifications banning irrational FDCs had been published in the *Gazette of India* and the industry could check the notifications online. The delegation was shell-shocked. Other associations also sought immediate meetings, and all of them were accommodated by the Ministry and apprised of the action taken. All associations were advised that there is no scope for any reversal of the decision. They were also persuaded to make a new beginning based on science and drop the idea of dragging the matter to the court as the step had been taken in the larger public interest.

There is an apprehension that some manufacturers did not apply for regularization of FDCs being manufactured by them. This suspicion arises from the fact that when a large delegation of pharmaceutical companies came for discussion after the ban on 344 FDCs was imposed in March 2016, one of the members asked how the government will deal with FDCs where the manufacturer forgot to submit the application for approval to the CDSCO.

The Minister met a delegation of Himachal Drug Manufacturers nearly after a month of the issuance of notifications prohibiting FDCs. In the meeting, the Minister assured that all possible assistance will be provided to the industry. He, however, made it clear that irrational drugs cannot be permitted to be sold in the market. In the meantime, the story was all over the print and electronic media. The media coverage largely appreciated the bold decision taken by the government; however, there were also some stories highlighting how the Indian pharmaceutical industry was hit badly by the sudden action of the government and without giving them an opportunity to put forth their view point.

MULTIPLE WRIT PETITIONS IN HIGH COURTS

A large number of writ petitions were filed in the Delhi High Court against the notifications prohibiting FDCs. Petitions were also filed in other High Courts across the country. The pharmaceutical industry engaged a battery of lawyers who comprised the who's who of the legal profession in India. In total, over 200 senior and other advocates appeared for the pharmaceutical companies in the Delhi High Court alone. After hearing the parties at length, the single learned Judge of the Delhi High Court concluded that prior consultation with the Drugs Technical Advisory Board (DTAB) set up under Section 5 of the Drugs & Cosmetics Act, 1940, was a condition precedent for exercising the power by the central government under Section 26A of the Drugs & Cosmetics Act, 1940.

In total, 505 petitions were disposed of by the Delhi High Court. This judgment was at variance with the judgments of the Karnataka and Madras High Courts, wherein those High Courts held that such consultation with the DTAB was not mandatory before exercise of power under Section 26A of the Drugs & Cosmetics Act, 1940.

SPECIAL LEAVE PETITION IN THE SUPREME COURT

The judgment of the Delhi High Court was examined by the MoHFW in consultation with the Ministry of Law & Justice, and a Special Leave Petition was filed in the Supreme Court against the order of the Delhi High Court. Petitions were also filed seeking transfer of all pending cases on the issue in all other High Courts to the Supreme Court. The transferred cases included those pending before the Madras High Court in respect of 294 FDC since 2007 referred to earlier. The Supreme Court, in its 54-page judgment, approved the two judgments of the Madras High Court and Karnataka High Court as having laid down the correct law on the construction of Section 26A of the Drugs & Cosmetics Act, 1940, namely that prior consultation with the DTAB was not mandatory for exercising powers vested in the central government. The judgments of the Delhi High Court were, accordingly, set aside. In the peculiar circumstances of the case, the Supreme Court gave further directions with a view to finding a science-based rational solution. The relevant extracts from the judgment of the Supreme Court are reproduced below for ready reference:

"32. On the facts of these cases, a suggested course of action was stated by learned counsel appearing on behalf of the petitioners/appellants. This course is that instead of now remitting the matter back to the Delhi High Court for an adjudication on the other points raised in the writ petitions, the case of 344 FDCs that have been banned, plus another 5 FDCs that have been banned, which comes to 349 FDCs, (barring 15 FDCs that are pre 1988 and 17 FDCs which have DCG(I) approval) pursuant to the Kokate Committee report, by notifications of the Central Government under Section 26A of the Drugs Act, should be sent to the DTAB, constituted under Section 5 of the Drugs Act, so that it can examine each of these cases and ultimately send a report to the Central Government. We reiterate that only on the peculiar facts of these cases, we think that such a course commends itself to us, which would obviate further litigation and finally set at rest all other contentions raised by the petitioners. We say so because we find that the Kokate Committee did deliberate on the 344 FDCs plus 5 FDCs and did come to a conclusion that the aforesaid FDCs be banned, but we are not clear as to what exactly the reasons for such conclusions are, and whether it was necessary in the public interest to take the extreme step of prohibiting such FDCs, instead of restricting or regulating their manufacture and supply. In order that an analysis be made in greater depth, we, therefore, feel that these cases should go to the DTAB and/or a Sub-Committee formed by the DTAB for the purpose of having a relook into these cases. It is important,

however, that the DTAB/Sub-Committee appointed for this purpose will not only hear the petitioners/appellants before us, but that they also hear submissions from the All India Drugs Action Network. The DTAB/Sub-Committee set up for this purpose will deliberate on the parameters set out in Section 26A of the Drugs Act, as follows.

33. First and foremost in each case, the DTAB/Sub-Committee appointed by it must satisfy itself that the use of the Fixed Dose Combinations (FDC) in question is likely to involve any one of the aforesaid three things: (a) that they are likely to involve any risk to human beings or animals; or (b) that the said FDCs do not have the therapeutic value claimed or purported to be claimed for them; or (c) that such FDCs contain ingredients and in such quantity for which there is no therapeutic justification.

34. The DTAB/Sub-Committee must also apply its mind as to whether it is then necessary or expedient, in the larger public interest, to regulate, restrict or prohibit the manufacture, sale or distribution of such FDCs. In short, the DTAB/Sub-Committee must clearly indicate in its report: (1) as to why, according to it, any one of the three factors indicated above is attracted; (2) post such satisfaction, that in the larger public interest, it is necessary or expedient to (i) regulate, (ii) restrict, or (iii) prohibit the manufacture, sale or distribution of such FDCs.

35. The DTAB/Sub-Committee must also indicate in its report as to why, in case it prohibits a particular FDC, restriction or regulation is not sufficient to control the manufacture and use of the FDC. We request the DTAB/Sub-Committee to be set up for this purpose to afford the necessary hearing to all concerned, and thereafter submit a consolidated report, insofar as these FDCs are concerned, to the Central Government within a period of six months from the date on which this judgment is received by the DTAB. We may also indicate that the Central Government, thereafter, must have due regard to the report of the DTAB and to any other relevant information, and ultimately apply its mind to the parameters contained in Section 26A of the Drugs Act and, accordingly, either maintain the notifications already issued, or modify/substitute them or withdraw them."[7]

CONSIDERATION BY DTAB SUB-COMMITTEE

In compliance of the Supreme Court directions, a sub-committee of the DTAB was constituted on 19.02.2018 for examining 349 FDCs under the Chairpersonship of Dr. Nilima Kshirsagar (Chair in Clinical Pharmacology, ICMR, Mumbai).The sub-committee's report was also accepted by the DTAB. It was submitted to the Ministry on 31.07.2018. After examination of the report, the Central Government again banned 328 FDCs and restricted the manufacture, sale or distribution of six FDCs subject to certain conditions on 07.09.2018. Further, 15 FDCs claimed to have been licensed prior to 1988 were not prohibited.

In compliance of the orders of the Supreme Court, the Sub-committee/DTAB and the government did all that was required to be done, and each of them applied themselves to the matter after affording necessary opportunity to all stakeholders. The sub-committee/DTAB had duly evaluated the risk involved and the therapeutic value and therapeutic justification for continuation or otherwise of the FDCs before making their recommendations to the central government.

BACK TO THE HIGH COURTS

Notwithstanding the verdict of the Supreme Court and the action taken by the government on the recommendations of the sub-committee of the DTAB and the DTAB itself, the manufacturers moved various High Courts again. In most cases, the High Courts had granted stay and some of the cases are still pending. It has been noted that in some cases, the High Courts are going into the merit of the decisions taken on the basis of

---

[7.] UNION OF INDIA, MINISTRY OF HEALTH AND FAMILY WELFARE *vs.* PFIZER LIMITED, available on https://main.sci.gov.in/case-status

science. As a consequence, the irrational FDCs that were permitted to be manufactured illegally by the state drug regulators continue to be marketed in the country, posing a risk to human lives.

While not sounding pessimistic, one would wonder whether after compliance with the Supreme Court directions in terms of examination of the merit or demerit of each FDC afresh by DTAB/its sub-committee and action taken by the government thereafter, could there have been any scope for further judicial scrutiny? One would be tempted to think that the judgment of the Supreme Court ought not to have been taken that lightly and the matter should not have been agitated afresh in the High Courts. Even if it be admitted that there was a scope for such a scrutiny, the marketing of such irrational FDCs should not have been permitted pending a final decision in the matter as the best technical experts in the field had, under the directions of the Supreme Court, categorically recommended those FDCs to be irrational/not justified. By granting the stay, the High Courts have opened the flood-gates for inflicting adverse impact of such FDCs on public health. In some cases, the High Courts have finally adjudicated the matter.

HONORING BOUNDARIES OF SCIENTIFIC KNOWLEDGE

One would have thought it appropriate to practice what Breyer Stephen said *"A judge is not a scientist, and a courtroom is not a scientific laboratory. But the law must seek decisions that fall within the boundaries of scientifically sound knowledge."*[8] In the present case, the science-based decisions taken by the government in accordance with the directions of the Supreme Court had been put on hold and the litigation continues.

It would, in this context, also be pertinent to refer to the following extracts from what the Delhi High Court had quoted in another case.[9]

[8.] Breyer, Stephen. "Science in the Courtroom." *Issues in Science and Technology* 16, no. 4 (Summer 2000).

[9.] W.P.(C) 6084/2018, C.M. APPL.23517/2018 BGP PRODUCTS OPERATIONS GMBH AND ANR versus UNION OF INDIA AND ORS

"Bernard Schwartz in Administrative Law, 2nd Edn., p. 584 has this to say about such function: 'If the scope of review is too broad, agencies are turned into little more than media for the transmission of cases to the courts. That would destroy the values of agencies created to secure the benefit of special knowledge acquired through continuous administration in complicated fields. At the same time, the scope of judicial inquiry must not be so restricted that it prevents full inquiry into the question of legality. If that question cannot be properly explored by the judge, the right to review becomes meaningless. It makes W.P.(C) 6084/2018 & connected matters judicial review of administrative orders a hopeless formality for the litigant.... It reduces the judicial process in such cases to a mere feint'".

There can be no doubt that the judiciary will continue to be expected to adjudicate scientific and technical issues; however, when an independent body comprising qualified technical personnel had examined the matter in pursuance of the directions of the Supreme Court, taking all scientific aspects into account, and made its recommendations on merit, judicial intervention should have been stopped. The judiciary might not be fully equipped to substitute the findings of technically qualified bodies based on scientific evidence by its own judgment based on technicalities and procedures. With due respect, it is considered that the intervention by various High Courts would, *prima facie,* appear to have been a case of judicial overreach in an area which might not be their *forte.*

In sum, the diffused responsibility orchestrated through a pre-independence legislation that is not fully in sync with the present constitutional mandate, presented a fertile field for some of the players in the pharmaceutical industry to make quick profits unabashedly with aggressive marketing, all the while conveniently ignoring public health concerns. Driven by greed, facilitated by legal loopholes and ably aided and propelled by the acquiescence or complacency of the drug regulatory structure in India, some players in the Indian pharmaceutical industry invented ways and means to frustrate any meaningful attempt to enforce regulation of FDCs in the country.

The dumping of FDCs in the most haphazard and unscientific manner in the Indian market without caring for the consequences, is a dark spot that has seriously compromised the current and future safety and health of patients and also damaged the reputation of the country. It could be nobody's case that the manufacturers of irrational and unapproved FDCs were not aware of the fact that some of these medicines are very powerful and, therefore, they should be used rationally in conformity with scientifically tested and approved pharmacological practices. There could also be no doubt that they were also aware of the fact that consumption of irrational FDCs in case of antibiotics will give rise to antimicrobial resistance that will make the most potent antibiotics of today redundant and future generations will be deprived of many useful antibiotics and their health benefits.

The actions of many FDC manufacturers, irresponsible as they were, posed serious challenge to human health. It also exposed the vulnerabilities of the archaic Drugs & Cosmetics Act, rules made there under and the incapacity of the government to take right decisions in the larger public interest under pressure from lobbies concerned. In the process, most pharmaceutical manufacturers in India continue to do what swell their profits with the least regard for science or for human health and welfare. What is astonishing is the fact that the entire system, bureaucracy, political executive and the judiciary has lent their support even if it is for technical or procedural reasons.

The question that needs to be pondered upon seriously is whether the profits of the pharmaceutical companies can be allowed to take precedence over public health of the present and future generations? The judiciary also needs to appreciate the point that clinical outcomes, effectiveness and appropriateness of medicines used to treat diseases, disorders and other health conditions need to be reviewed from time to time through science-based evidence, and any approval given in the past even by the competent authorities has to be subject to review based on such further evidence as emerges with the new scientific developments and knowledge. Keeping that in view, even the decision of the judiciary to permit manufacture of FDCs that had been approved by DCG(I) but were now found to be irrational based on scientific knowledge that become available over time, is questionable. We will do well to remember that *salus populi suprema lex esto* or the good of the people is the supreme law and no one, not even the courts of law, should interfere when an action is taken for the welfare of the people, least of all for technical or procedural reasons.

CHAPTER 6

MAKING SENSE OF THE POLICY-MAKING CONUNDRUM

The previous chapter, *inter alia*, mentioned how the art of not making decisions has been perfected by the bureaucratic structures. It narrated how a seasoned public administrator invariably looks for a way out for deferring the decision when taking one is not convenient. The advantages of not taking the bull by its horns may be many but that option may not be available in all circumstances. The useful and the oft-practiced trick of constituting a committee or a group could buy some time, but not always. The chapter encapsulated how, initially the inaction or timid action and later, the technicalities and procedural issues ensured the continued marketing of irrational FDCs without bothering about the cost that it could entail in terms of human and animal health. The major highlight of the chapter was that the political executive was largely neutral and did not interfere with the processes, but also did not shy away from taking a decision that was appropriate in the circumstances.

This chapter seeks to make sense of the policy making conundrum in the Indian context, especially when the political executive gets into an overdrive and makes efforts to hijack public policy without appreciating the scientific rationale, and persists with the beliefs and practices borne out of their roles as activists. With the senior-most bureaucrats still seeking to wriggle out as long as that is possible, the officials at the cutting edge are left to bear the burden. The three issues covered in this chapter are: regulation of oxytocin, its manufacturing, sale and misuse in India; the *Pradhan Mantri Bhartiya Jan Aushadhi Pariyojna* and the rationalization of customs duty on drugs. These highlight three different genres of perils associated with decision making in the government.

REGULATION OF OXYTOCIN

Maneka Sanjay Gandhi[1] is a known animal rights activist and is a vociferous propagator of the cause of animals. Be it the misuse of oxytocin or use of animals in the testing of cosmetics and drugs, she has continued to spearhead the crusade to further the rights of animals. In the process, very often, she could get on one's nerves if and when she finds the person standing in her way. It would generally be a difficult task to change her views. In such circumstances, most officials adopt the strategy of keeping the discussion with her on different issues to the bare minimum. Many of them would not prefer to explain persuasively and with conviction the rationale or the reason as to why what Mrs. Gandhi wanted to be done is not in the larger public interest. At the same time, while not giving up the cause, she would generally be open to interim solutions as long as those helped in furthering the cause being pursued by her. However, when the officials are not forthcoming with convincing alternatives, the position taken by her can only harden and it would not matter if it is harmful to the cause of humans. She would not hesitate to use her stature to bulldoze things around and, very often, the starting point in her conversations could be the one of putting the person she is communicating with on the defensive.

The alleged misuse of oxytocin on cows purportedly for letting the milk down quickly and its use for quick growth of vegetable and fruits is one issue which has been pursued by her aggressively. In July 2014, Mrs. Gandhi mentioned that the MoHFW was taking no concrete action for banning oxytocin and also for banning testing of cosmetic products on animals. She continued to pursue these matters with all officials concerned and told them that the Ministry was not bothered about the subject and cows were being subjected to unwarranted cruelty. Pointing out that the details available with the Ministry did not make out a case for prohibition of oxytocin and that the related issues had been considered a number of times in the Drug Technical Advisory Board, examined on file and that it

[1.] Maneka Sanjay Gandhi is an Indian politician, animal rights activist and environmentalist. She is a Member of Parliament and has held various positions in the Government of India, including that of a Cabinet Minister in the Union government.

was, *inter alia*, being used in managing postpartum cases, did not cut ice with Mrs. Gandhi. She was also informed that the studies conducted by the National Institute of Nutrition, ICMR and other government institutes did not reveal that oxytocin was harmful to animals.

Not satisfied with the argument, she convened a meeting in her office in which all senior officials of the MoHFW were present. Surprisingly, most of the senior officials did not speak a word other than exchanging pleasantries and listened to what she had to say. However, the then DGHS informed her that since the drug has a therapeutic value, its banning was not the solution. Mrs. Gandhi handed over photocopies of some studies indicating the harmful effects of oxytocin and told the DGHS that he was blissfully ignorant on the issue and desired that the MoHFW should, keeping in view the findings of those studies, take urgent action to ban oxytocin. On perusal of the reports handed over by her, it was noticed that those pertained to some innocuous studies undertaken in Pakistan and not in any developed country and, moreover, the papers had not been published in any journal of repute.

RESTRICTING OXYTOCIN MANUFACTURING TO A SINGLE PSU

After some days, Mrs. Gandhi deputed her Private Secretary (PS) to discuss the pending issues of concern to animals in the Ministry of Health and Family Welfare. In the meeting it was clearly told that in the given circumstances, the best that was possible was to take action against the illicit/illegal manufacturing and use of oxytocin and its other concoctions, but banning it was not possible. The issue of restricting manufacturing of oxytocin to a single PSU was also discussed for reducing its misuse. The Minister's PS was advised that this issue was not within the remit of the MoHFW and, in any case, it would require approval of the Cabinet since it will be an alteration of the country's industrial policy and creating a monopoly could create problems in the availability of and access to oxytocin.

Mrs. Gandhi later informed that she was not in favor of taking the matter to the Cabinet and it may be settled at a departmental level. She deputed her Officer on Special Duty (OSD) and a couple of other staff to pursue a few other matters, including use of animals for testing of cosmetics. Mrs. Gandhi had also spoken to the then Minister of Health and Family Welfare, J P Nadda, and also Secretary, MoHFW. She continued to pursue the matter with the Health Minister almost during or after every meeting of the Cabinet.

The Health Minister made sincere efforts to find a solution to the issue being flagged by Mrs. Gandhi and convened a meeting to discuss the issue in his office. It was decided in the meeting that in view of the insistence of Mrs. Gandhi, a meeting could be called at Secretary Level in which Secretary, Department of Industrial Policy and Promotion, and Secretary, Department of Pharmaceuticals could also be invited. The issue was discussed, but no progress could be made in the matter in the meeting. Another meeting was convened by Mrs. Gandhi in her office in Shastri Bhawan in which she expressed her anguish on the points raised by the then Secretary, Department of Pharmaceuticals.

MARKETING OF ILLEGAL OXYTOCIN CONCOCTION

Keeping in view the widespread misuse of oxytocin for veterinary use, restrictions had already been placed on use of Oxytocin under the Drugs & Cosmetics Rules, 1945. The sale of oxytocin injection had been placed under Schedule 'H' of the Drugs & Cosmetics Rules, 1945.[2] It required the drug to be dispensed only on the prescription of a Registered Medical Practitioner and its packaging was permitted only in a single unit blister pack to avoid misuse.

To curb the misuse of oxytocin, its manufacture for sale or for distribution and sale was restricted further in January 2014. In accordance with the restriction, the manufacturers of bulk oxytocin could supply the active pharmaceutical ingredient of oxytocin only to the manufacturers licensed under the Drugs and Cosmetics Rules, 1945 for manufacturing

---

[2.] Schedule 'H' contains details of the drugs that can be sold only on the prescription of a Registered Medical Practitioner.

its formulations. The formulations meant for veterinary use could, as per the restriction, be sold only to veterinary hospitals. The restrictions did, however, not make much of a difference as there was inadequate machinery for enforcement at the field level and it was not geared to take on the task. This aspect also needs to be seen in the light of the limited role of the CDSCO and the central government in drug regulation and the unwillingness of the state governments and regulators to cooperate in such matters.

In June 2015, Mrs. Maneka Sanjay Gandhi sent a dozen bottles labeled as oxytocin in 250 ml plastic packs, bought by her staff from the outskirts of Delhi, to the MoHFW as evidence of the extensive misuse of oxytocin. The Minister highlighted the misuse of the drug and enquired whether in view of the solid evidence having been provided, the Ministry would ban manufacturing and marketing of oxytocin. While informing Mrs. Gandhi that banning the drug would not be feasible, it was indicated that best possible efforts will be made to curb the misuse of the drug for veterinary purposes. The samples of the concoction were sent to the Central Drug Laboratory, Kolkata for tests and analysis. It was found that these samples contained oxytocin with large number of impurities.

After enquiries, it was found that there was no manufacturing facility at the addresses printed on the labels of the samples. Thereafter, some surprise checks were undertaken to collect legal samples to initiate action under the Drugs & Cosmetics Act, 1940. The inspectors of the CDSCO, North Zone, picked up samples from areas in the vicinity of dairies in East, South West and North Delhi from dairies and vendors who were selling the concoction. This corroborated the view of Mrs. Maneka Gandhi that there was a widespread and clandestine misuse of oxytocin in the dairy industry.

Further inquiries were conducted by the CDSCO officials who were able to trace some of the manufacturers. Their manufacturing facilities were raided and serious lapses were detected. It was noticed that many manufacturers were not licensed and were mixing oxytocin API with water in the open and packing it for use in dairy and other industries.

Simultaneously, efforts continued to be made to locate the source from where the oxytocin active pharmaceutical ingredient had been bought.

A CDSCO team had earlier been deputed to ascertain whether the only bulk supplier in India had made the API available to any unlicensed manufacturers. From the documents inspected, the CDSCO team concluded that no such supplies had been made by that firm to unlicensed manufacturers. Further, surveillance was launched at different places, including at various airports and sea ports in close cooperation with customs authorities.

MEETING IN PMO AND FOLLOW-UP ACTION

In the meantime, the matter was escalated by Mrs. Gandhi to the level of the Principal Secretary to the Prime Minister, who convened a meeting on 26.09.2015 in which a number of decisions were taken. In pursuance of the decisions taken in the PMO meeting, a multipronged approach was adopted by CDSCO to unearth the clandestine manufacture, import and distribution of oxytocin. Several teams comprising officials from the CDSCO and independent persons not associated with the government were constituted to spearhead investigations into illegal import, export and domestic supplies of raw materials and finished products of oxytocin at various air and sea ports.

Based on the preliminary information gathered by the CDSCO, it was decided to keep a close vigil on M/s Fedex Express Transportation and Supply Chain Services (India) Pvt. Ltd., Mayapuri Industrial Area, New Delhi – a courier company through which oxytocin was allegedly being imported under the name of Custom Peptide. After four days of constant vigil and coordinated efforts, the CDSCO team nabbed one individual who hailed from Kolkata in the premises of M/s Fedex in Mayapuri Industrial Area, New Delhi on 30.10.2015 when he had gone to the Fedex office and received the imported consignments of Custom Peptide.

On being confronted, the individual disclosed the names of three persons and locations in Kolkata, Patna and Ludhiana where oxytocin under the name of Custom Peptide was allegedly being supplied illegally.

In the meantime, the sample of Custom Peptide was drawn from one of the consignments from Fedex premises and tested and analyzed at the Indian Pharmacopoeia Commission Laboratory, Ghaziabad. The tests and analysis revealed the content to be pure oxytocin.

Three special teams comprising officers of the CDSCO were constituted to undertake investigation at three locations disclosed by the said individual. The first team led by the Joint Drug Controller conducted an investigation in a premises at Kolkata, along with West Bengal state drugs control officials, Kolkata Police, Anti-Corruption Wings of the CBI and the Narcotic Control Bureau (NCB). The state police and other state authorities deliberately delayed the CDSCO team from reaching the location of the alleged manufacturing of oxytocin from imported peptide on the ground of jurisdiction of the police station.

During investigation, the team observed that white powder and liquid (purported to be oxytocin) and narcotic drugs were stocked at the said premises. Subsequently, the stock was seized by the CDSCO officials and the narcotic drugs were seized by the officers of Narcotics Control Bureau (NCB) under Narcotic Drugs & Psychotropic Substances Act, 1985. While the owner of the house was arrested, the kingpin of the entire process managed to flee. Scrutiny of documents revealed that no license had been obtained either to manufacture or store pharmaceutical products in that premises.

The second team of the CDSCO along with officials from State Drug Control Authority, Punjab jointly conducted surprise inspections on the wholesale premises of one medical store in Ludhiana and its owner's residence on 31.10.2015 and 01.11.2015. However, the team could not lay its hands on any evidence about the illegal sale of oxytocin in this case. The team also conducted surprise inspections of four licensed chemist shops suspected of selling oxytocin injections to dairy owners in Ludhiana. In one of the shops on Tajpur Road, Ludhiana, the team seized 67 unlabeled bottles suspected to be oxytocin injection and 16 bottles labeled as 'Oxytocin Injection Veterinary'.

The third team of CDSCO along with the state drug control officials of Bihar conducted joint raids at three places in Patna on 31.10.2015 and 01.11.2015. Two licensed firms having the same name were raided simultaneously as these were reported to be involved in illegal manufacture of oxytocin. While no evidence was available in one case, in another premises, the team observed that the firm was not complying with most of the requirements of GMP as per Schedule 'M' of the Drugs & Cosmetics, Rules, 1945 for manufacturing oxytocin injection. The team filed a complaint at Khajekala Police Station, Patna City.

The CDSCO also asked the Bihar's state drug controller to provide a list of licensed oxytocin manufacturers. The state drug controller took a lot of time to supply the information as the information was reportedly not available. The list showed that a large number of manufacturers were located in Gaya. The CDSCO deputed three teams to Gaya for undertaking unscheduled inspection of the oxytocin manufacturers. The inspections brought out that none of the drug manufacturing plants inspected had any semblance of complying with the GMP.

In one particular case, it was revealed that the manufacturing unit was located in a narrow lane that could be reached only by a two-wheeler. In the premises where the drugs were being manufactured, the ground floor housed cows and buffaloes, the first floor had the manufacturing unit and the top floor was being used as the residence of the owner. In the name of GMP, there was only a pedestal fan and active pharmaceuticals were lying scattered on the floor. So much for GMP! Earlier, after receiving the news of inspection, the front side of the unit had been closed. The inspection team managed to enter from the back gate, which was open as it was also the way to the residence on the top floor. FIRs were registered against the manufacturers. The inspection team also noted that besides the licensed manufacturers, there were a number of unlicensed manufacturers operating illegally in Gaya.

LITIGATION IN THE HIGH COURT OF HIMACHAL PRADESH

In a separate development, the matter relating to abuse of oxytocin had been taken up for examination by the High Court of Himachal Pradesh.

In its order dated 15.3.2016, the Himachal High Court gave directions to, *inter alia*, establish an efficient drug regulatory system, both at the Centre and the state, for better co-ordination and handling matters concerning regulation of the manufacture, import and distribution, especially of drugs such as oxytocin; consider the feasibility of restricting the manufacture of oxytocin to a single PSU and also restricting and limiting the manufacturing of oxytocin by companies to whom licenses had already been granted.

The judgment bolstered the case for restricting the manufacturing of oxytocin to a single Public Sector Unit (PSU), and Mrs. Gandhi and her team became very active. Mrs. Gandhi forwarded a copy of the order of the Himachal High Court to the MoHFW and advised immediate steps to be taken for restricting the manufacturing of oxytocin to a single PSU.

On examination, it was pointed out that imposing such a restriction was not in consonance with the government's policy; such an action will restrict the sources of supply, leading to a monopoly situation and it could also create price instability. It was also pointed out that since this did not form part of the mandate of the MoHFW under the Government of Indian (Allocation of Business) Rules, 1961, it would be beyond the competence of the Ministry to take any such decision and, therefore, the matter should be examined by the Departments concerned. It was also highlighted that the capacity of the PSU proposed by the Department of Pharmaceuticals to take up the manufacturing was not adequate to meet the country's requirements.

In a meeting held in the MoHFW, it was concluded that any such restriction will be disastrous and not in keeping with the government's policy of minimum government, maximum governance. On the contrary, it was informed that the problem could be resolved by strengthening the drug regulatory structures in the country to curb the misuse of drugs and also for improving the quality of drugs through better regulation. In the meantime, the clamp down on the illegal import, manufacturing and sale of oxytocin was intensified.

CHANGE IN THE STANCE OF THE HEALTH MINISTRY

Things changed with the passage of time, especially after the abrupt changes in the senior management in the MoHFW in June 2017. The pressure for implementation of the Order of the Himachal High Court intensified, culminating in the Notification dated 27.04.2018, which was later impugned in the Delhi High Court. The Delhi High Court in its reasoned judgment[3] held that the impugned notification was both unreasonable and arbitrary and the government had not adequately weighed the danger to the users of oxytocin nor considered the deleterious effect to the public generally and particularly the pregnant women and young mothers, of the possible restricted supply if manufacture of a lifesaving drug was confined to one unit.

The Delhi High Court held that the risk of such an action can be drastic; the scarcity of the drug or even its restricted availability can increase maternal fatalities during childbirth, impairing lives of thousands of innocent mothers. The impugned notification and all the consequential orders were declared arbitrary and unreasonable by the Delhi High Court and were, therefore, quashed and set aside.[4]

The matter did not end with the Delhi High Court judgment as the judgments of the Himachal High Court and the Delhi High Court were contradictory. The Central Government filed an appeal against Delhi HC judgment in the matter before the Supreme Court. The Division Bench of the Supreme Court referred the matter to a larger bench as in opinion of the court, it raised serious issues with far-reaching implications.

This case manifests the inability of the governmental structures to look out for the root cause of the problem and evolve appropriate solutions in the light of interference by the political executive. In this case, the basic principle of first defining the problem and then evolving solutions had

---

3. All India Drug Action Network v. Union of India and Anr. WP(C) 8555/2018, clubbed with WP (C) 2084/2018, 8666/2018 and 9601/2018. 2018 Dec 4 [cited 2019 Mar 11]. Available on: http://lobis.nic.in/ddir/dhc/SRB/judgement/14-12-2018/ SRB14122018CW60842018.pdf

4. WP (C) 2084/2018, 8666/2018 and 9601/2018. 2018 Dec 4 [cited 2019 Mar 11]. Available at: http://lobis.nic.in/ddir/dhc/SRB/judgement/14-12-2018/

been given a farewell, and the extraneous solutions without considering their pros and cons were sought to be implemented. As would be evident from the details brought out in this book, the root cause of the problem lies in the absence of adequate regulation by a diffused regulatory structure in an environment where some operators have hijacked the system with the sole objective of minting profits at the cost of the larger public good.

PRADHAN MANTRI BHARTIYA JAN AUSHADHI PARIYOJNA

The second stance of poor policy making is the *Pradhan Mantri Bhartiya Jan Aushadhi Pariyojna*[5] (PMBJP) which, in its new *avatar*, has been touted as the game changer. The scheme was launched in 2008 with the objective of making quality medicines available at affordable prices for all, particularly the poor and the disadvantaged sections of society through exclusive outlets. The rationale for the scheme was to reduce the out-of-pocket expenses related to healthcare, ostensibly due to the high cost of branded drugs in India. The intent of PMBJP is noble; however, the scheme is structured on a faulty understanding of the ground realities, and there are serious gaps in the scheme and its implementation.

The government claims that the scheme has, in its revamped format, increased the bouquet of medicines being sold through these stores with no stock outs and substantial increase in the number of PMBJP stores. The medicines, as per the claims, are being sold at prices that are 50% to 90% cheaper as compared with market prices and 90% lesser vis-à-vis the prices of branded medicines. The claim also goes on to add that the medicines supplied by the PMBJP stores are WHO-GMP and NABL certified.

The central government has recognized that the scheme was largely a failure till 2012–13, with limited reach through a handful of outlets; limited medicines being sold through these stores; and frequent stock outs. The ground reality even in respect of the revamped scheme is, however,

---

[5] The scheme was earlier known as *Jan Aushadhi* Scheme. It was rechristened as *Pradhan Mantri Bharatiya Jan Aaushadhi Pariyojana* (PMBJP) two years after the NDA government took over in 2014.

no different. There are serious concerns with regard to the quality and availability of medicines at the PMBJP stores. The concerns relate to non-transparent procurement processes and also the quality of medicines, including the testing procedures adopted before procurement from new vendors with no track record of having supplied quality medicines.

More than 50% of the drugs procured, as reported under the PMBJP scheme, are stated to be slow-moving. As per reports appearing in the print media, drugs past their expiry dates were also being sold at some PMBJP stores.

The stance taken by the government in this case is misleading in so far as its references to the branded and generic medicines are concerned. India is not known for branded drugs and most branded drugs are imported. Largely, generic medicines are marketed in India and the branded drugs certainly do not cater to the poor and the disadvantaged sections of the society. Therefore, the question of high cost of branded drugs affecting the poor is absurd.

An important aspect that cannot be ignored is that the generic medicines manufactured in India are not of uniform quality[6] and the insistence of the government only on generic names being put on the label of the medicines or prescription of medicines only by generic names is arbitrary and illogical. Such an unreasonable restriction impedes the autonomy of the consumer in making a well-considered choice. It brackets the medicines of good quality that meet all requirements, including stability, bioequivalence, dissolution, etc., with those which might only be pharmaceutically equivalent.

There are a large number of manufacturers who comply with neither the GMP specified in the Drugs & Cosmetics Rules, 1945 nor WHO-GMP, as revealed by the risk-based inspections undertaken by the CDSCO.[7] Further, a very large number of unlicensed pharmaceutical manufacturers still continue to manufacture drugs in India and a number of manufacturing units only manufacture for government supplies and operate only when they have bagged an order. Medicines manufactured by them are also labeled as generic medicines.

[6.] For details refer to the findings of the largest ever drug survey detailed in Chapter 4.
[7.] For details refer to the findings of Risk Based Inspections detailed in Chapter 4.

Neither the WHO nor the NABL certify the quality of medicines and the government's claim in that regard is ridiculous. PMBJP needs to be viewed in the context of the larger prevalence of poor-quality medicines in government supplies. It is strange that the government has, at the highest level, been propagating the scheme without caring about concerns regarding the quality of the drugs. In a communication sent to the Prime Minister's Office in 2016, the MoHFW had advised that all generics are not of the same quality and, therefore, the labeling requirements that insist only on using the generic names could be problematic and the PMBJP schemes needs to be looked at *de novo*.

This case reflects that the bureaucracy including its technical part, are not in a position to advise the political leadership appropriately. This is akin to the situation narrated in the story *The Emperor's New Clothes,* in which no body is ready to tell the king that he is naked for the fear of losing his position or being labeled stupid. It is also a clear case of playing to the gallery at some cost to public health.

To any unbiased and prudent observer of the pharmaceutical sector, PMBJP would appear to be morally suspect sales tactics that are unwittingly also being promoted by the government. Such governmental support helps in luring customers to buy pharmaceutical products with suspect claims. The gravy train that facilitates making money quickly and through means that might not be above board should not have been sponsored by the government. It needs to be noted that the current policy of damn the torpedoes could have serious public health consequences.

RATIONALIZING CUSTOMS DUTY

The Department of Revenue was keen on removing the existing customs duty concessions wherever feasible with a view to enhance revenue receipts. With this objective, it had been pursuing the MoHFW and the Department of Pharmaceuticals to suggest drugs where the concessions provided for levying customs duty could be withdrawn in view of the domestic production facilities having been established. Both the MoHFW and the

Department of Pharmaceuticals had, based on an exercise undertaken by them separately communicated the list of such drugs to the Department of Revenue. However, the Department of Pharmaceuticals later withdrew their list for unexplained reasons.

In a notification of 28.01.2016, the Department of Revenue, Ministry of Finance removed the customs duty exemption for 76 drugs where domestic manufacturing had commenced. While most of the print media was comparatively restrained in its criticism and, in some cases, accommodated the government viewpoint, others especially the electronic media came out with imaginative stories of how the prices of lifesaving drugs will shoot up by as much as 35%. It became a matter of heated debate on the prime-time television channels for weeks, together with all kinds of arguments being furthered by participants for and against the move depending upon which side of the fence the participant belonged to. In general, the electronic media decried the decision of the government and elected to play to the gallery and portrayed the decision – allegedly taken in pursuance of the 'Make in India' objective – as anti-patient.

The response of the pharmaceutical industry associations was nuanced and the Indian Drug Manufacturers Association and Indian Pharmaceutical Alliance, the two leading associations of drug manufacturing companies, supported the decision of the government, giving detailed reasons for it. The only exception to this was Kiran Mazumder-Shaw of Biocon, who vehemently opposed the withdrawal of customs duty concessions. Later, in a meeting in the MoHFW, the Biocon founder explained that the notifications will hit her products as her manufacturing facilities were located in a Special Economic Zone. She was very agitated about it when she was apprised that the entire matter had been reviewed by the government and the product being manufactured by her company will not be getting the exemption back. The companies had to absorb the additional cost as the products formed part of the National List of Essential Medicines and was subject to price control under the DPCO.

The incessant media criticism and the arguments put forward by many stakeholders forced the Prime Minister's Office (PMO) to convene a meeting with the Secretaries of the Departments of Revenue, Pharmaceutical, and Health and Family Welfare. Surprisingly, in the very first meeting, the Department of Revenue, who had issued the notification, disowned the decision and informed that the notification withdrawing customs duty had been issued after consultation with the MoHFW and the Department of Pharmaceuticals.

After the meetings in the PMO, the then Secretary, Health and Family Welfare panicked and enquired whether he had seen the file. He was apprised that since it was only information sharing and the decision had to be taken by the Department of Revenue it did not require approval at Secretary level. That information relieved him.

The Principal Secretary to the Prime Minister convened another meeting the following Saturday to discuss the issue. As informed by another senior officer present in the meeting in the PMO, Secretary, Health and Family Welfare repeatedly highlighted that the decision to share the information with the Department of Revenue had been taken by the Joint Secretary at his level and the Secretary was not in the picture. His entire effort was to ensure that he should not be held blameworthy for any decision in the matter.

It goes to the credit of the then Principal Secretary to the PM that he categorically told that it did not matter at which level the decision had been taken and that the three departments must examine the impact of the decision objectively and a group of officers of the three departments should undertake the exercise within the next three to four days. He pointed out that decisions could go wrong and if they do, necessary corrective action should be taken rather than finding fault.

As decided in the aforesaid meeting, the group comprising Joint Secretary (R), MoHFW; Joint Secretary, Pharmaceuticals; Member Secretary, National Pharmaceuticals Pricing Authority; and a representative of the Department of Revenue examined the matter on the basis of data collected by the NPPA and the CDSCO. The officials of the NPPA and CDSCO worked day and night to dig out the relevant data about imports, prices of bulk drugs, prices of formulations and other ingredients, etc., for three days. The group assessed the impact of the decision on the availability and price of each medicine.

In order to validate the findings, the group also had detailed discussions with Heads of Departments/senior doctors from the relevant specialties from AIIMS, New Delhi, Ram Manohar Lohia and Safdarjung Hospitals, New Delhi. The group assessed that the impact on either the availability of medicines or their prices would be negligible in all cases, except for four medicines. They recommended that withdrawal of the customs duty waiver could be rolled back as far as these four drugs were concerned as sanctioned capacity had not been utilized for various reasons.

Secretary, Health and Family Welfare further checked the position about the four drugs from different sources, including the Heads of Department in AIIMS, New Delhi, who supported the recommendations of the group. In respect of one drug, it was opined that the indigenous products were good and if the customs duty waiver is not revived, it will lead to the growth of the domestic industry. Keeping in view the fact that licensed capacity for manufacturing Octreotide, used generally to treat hormonal disorders; Somatropin used for treatment of growth failure and Anti-haemophilic factor concentrate (VIII & IX) was not being fully, the customs duty exemption was restored.

The case highlights the unwillingness of the bureaucratic structures to make decisions due to the fear of being hauled up.

Together, the three cases highlight the perils of decision making in the government and portray how on occasions, extraneous considerations and on others, inability to stand by those who take decisions, impact policy making. In some instances, the policy-makers also play to the gallery rather than look at the real gain from decisions made and senior bureaucrats fret to find ways to save their skin.

CHAPTER 7

POST MARKETING SURVEILLANCE

It is well acknowledged that for all medicines there is a trade-off between the benefits and the potential for harm. A fairly good part of the discussion in this book so far has concerned the quality and safety of drugs. Continuing the same, this chapter captures another dimension relating to continued assessment of the safety of drugs over a longer period of time after they enter the market. The chapter assesses the current position of post marketing surveillance in India.

Though a drug undergoes extensive screening before its approval, it is not possible to capture all adverse drug reactions (ADRs) as clinical trials are often small, short and invariably biased. The clinical trials generally do not include patients with co-morbid diseases, pregnant women, children and elderly as participants. In the clinical trials, most drugs are tested only for short-term safety and efficacy on a limited number of carefully selected individuals, which could be anywhere between a few hundred to a few thousand. Pre-marketing trials cannot, therefore, mirror actual clinical use situations in view of factors such as diverse ethnicity and non-representative character of trial participants. It is, in this scenario, not possible to identify or detect all possible ADRs during trials. No doubt, many adverse effects, interactions with different foods or other medicines and other unknown risks come to light over a period time, sometimes years after the medical product has been in use. Such ADRs impact the quality of life, result in prolonged hospitalization and increase mortality.

Monitoring the quality, safety and efficacy of a medicine throughout its use for treatment is, therefore, important. A decision regarding continuation or otherwise of a medical product for treatment has to be taken on the basis of a careful analysis of the risks involved and the potential benefit coming to light over a longer period of time. Post marketing surveillance (PMS) is, as such, a very important part of drug development and plays a crucial role for deciding continued use of a drug. PMS activities are mandatory under the Drugs & Cosmetics Rules, 1945. With effect from March 2016, establishment of the pharmacovigilance system and appointment of a qualified officer to manage it has also been made mandatory for better surveillance of medical products.

PHARMACOVIGILANCE

Early detection of the possible risks associated with the use of drugs through systematic approach for PMS or pharmacovigilance constitutes a critical element of the regulatory framework. PMS is a very helpful tool for perfecting new processes for better analysis of the risk-benefit ratio of drugs. It is an integral part of drug discovery and development, and is primarily designed to collect and collate information about the safety of a drug after it has been placed in the market. It provides information to the regulator about any adverse event associated with the use of a drug, including amongst those who had been exposed to the drug during clinical trials and also about adverse drug reactions that were ascertained during its usage in clinical practices.

WHO defines pharmacovigilance as the science and activities relating to detection, assessment, understanding and prevention of adverse effects or any other possible drug-related problems.[1] It also includes gathering information about substandard medicines, medication errors, lack of efficacy reports, use of medicines for indications that are not approved and for which there is inadequate scientific basis, case reports of acute and chronic poisoning, assessment of drug-related mortality, abuse and misuse of medicines, adverse interactions of medicines with chemicals, other medicines and food, etc. Pharmacovigilance, as such, acts as an important

---

[1.] The IMPORTANCE of PHARMACOVIGILANCE Safety Monitoring of medicinal products' 2002

surveillance mechanism to monitor the safety and promotes rational use of medicines.

The origin of pharmacovigilance can be traced to the death of Hannah in 1848 due to chloroform. Though formal process of pharmacovigilance was initiated after the reporting of the unfortunate thalidomide disaster of 1961/62[2] in which over 10,000 children in 46 countries were born with birth defects on account of use of a substandard quality drug, Thalidomide. The drug had been introduced in Germany in 1957 and was widely prescribed for treatment of morning sickness and nausea in pregnant women. When it was found that babies of women using Thalidomide were born without limbs, its use was discontinued. It was in the aftermath of this tragedy that WHO started a pilot research project for International Drug Monitoring in 1968 with a view to developing a system for detecting previously unknown or poorly understood adverse effects of medicines.

WHO lists out the aims of pharmacovigilance as improving patient care and safety in relation to the use of medicines and all medical and paramedical interventions, improve public health and safety, contribute to the assessment of benefit, harm, effectiveness and risk of medicines, thus encouraging their safe, rational and more effective use, and promoting the understanding, education and clinical training in pharmacovigilance and its effective communication to the public.[3]

As a dynamic scientific discipline, pharmacovigilance helps in minimizing the harm from the use of medicines and also helps in initiating necessary corrective action where required. It also acts as an important enabler for ensuring that medicines of good quality that are safe and efficacious only are used and that too rationally, while taking the expectations and concerns of patients into account when therapeutic decisions are made. It helps in minimizing the risk of harm by keeping the health professionals informed. Communicating such adverse effects

---

[2.] Fora tabular representation of the milestones in the journey of pharmacovigilance, see https://link.springer.com/article/10.1007/s11096-018-0657-1/figures/1.

[3.] https://apps.who.int/Iris/bitstream/handle/10665/42493/a75646.pdf

and toxicity associated with the medicine not noticed previously to those who are responsible for appropriate action, is important for initiating the necessary corrective steps.

With over one-sixth of the humanity residing in India and as the largest producer of generic medicines globally, India needs robust monitoring structures to ensure that only the best-quality drugs are marketed. Keeping in view the fact that the quality of healthcare facilities varies from region to region, the Indian population would encounter ADRs distinct from those noticed in other countries. Even within India, the ADRs could differ to some extent on account of differences in ethnicity. This calls for establishment of a robust techno-science-based system for monitoring ADRs. The outcomes, such as the safety of medicines, lower morbidity and mortality, reduced period of hospitalization and lower treatment costs, are some of the benefits of pharmacovigilance. It is a useful tool for disease surveillance, including in pandemic-like situations and could be the key to evolving solutions for disease control.

PHARMACOVIGILANCE PROGRAM OF INDIA

Even though the Indian pharmaceutical industry expanded very fast during the last three decades, the evolution of regulatory structures and practices was much slower. For example, the Pharmacovigilance Program of India (PvPI) was initiated only in 2010. The responsibility for this program was initially entrusted to the All India Institute of Medical Sciences (AIIMS), New Delhi, which was made the National Coordinating Centre for monitoring ADRs in the country. However, subsequently, with a view to scale up the activities, the National Coordination Centre was shifted from AIIMS, New Delhi to the Indian Pharmacopoeia Commission, Ghaziabad in April 2011. The mandate of the PvPI includes creation of a nation-wide system for ensuring patient safety through better ADRs reporting; to identify and analyze new signals on ADRs from reported cases; to analyze the benefit–risk ratio of marketed medications; to support regulatory agencies in the decision-making process regarding use of medications; to communicate the safety information relating to the use of medicines to various stakeholders with a view to minimize risks; to collaborate with national centers of other countries for exchanging information and data management; and to provide training and consultancy support to other pharmacovigilance centers globally. The PvPI safeguards the health of human beings by ensuring that the benefit of use of medicine outweighs the risks associated with its use.

The PvPI, after its location in the Indian Pharmacopoeia Commission, has expanded very fast. At the end of July 2020, the PvPI had established 311 ADR Monitoring Centers (AMCs) across the country to monitor and report ADRs. ADR reporting is taking place through helpline and mobile apps. Even patients can report events directly. The ADRs reported to PvPI are processed, and alerts and interventions are generated and transmitted to all concerned automatically.

The PvPI has put in place a robust mechanism, and has engaged dedicated human resources at recognized AMCs, both in the public and the private sector to boost pharmacovigilance practices. Also, AMC focal persons along with their teams have continued to be trained and provided with technical guidelines, ADRs reporting tools and other accessories for seamless functioning. All recognized AMCs have been enabled to submit Individual Case Safety Reports (ICSRs) through VigiFlow.[4] PvPI has also been partnering with Marketing Authorization Holders (MAHs) of pharmaceutical products and professional bodies such as the Indian Medical Association, Indian Pharmacological Society and others. Based on the analysis of ICSRs, the PvPI identifies safety signals and provides recommendations about regulatory action required to be taken by the CDSCO. Local ADR Monitoring Centers (AMCs) have been co-located with medical institutions. The ICSRs collected by PvPI are also shared with the global database of adverse drug reactions, namely Vigibase

---

[4.] VigiFlow is a management system for recording, processing and sharing reports of adverse effects. It supports domestic collection and processing of individual case safety report data. (https://www.who-umc.org/global-pharmacovigilance/vigiflow)

hosted by Uppsala Monitoring Centre (UMC), under the aegis of the WHO.

The broadened patient safety scope of pharmacovigilance includes detection of medicines of substandard quality, as well as prescribing, dispensing and administration errors. Counterfeiting, antimicrobial resistance[5] and real-time surveillance in mass vaccinations are the other pharmacovigilance challenges that need to be addressed.

The PvPI conducts a number of training programs, both for the public and private sectors to enable clarity about basic concepts. Such programs help in understanding the system of ADR reporting, use of tools and methods, causality assessment, regulatory pharmacovigilance and signal detection. Technical expertise available in both public and private sectors has continued to be utilized for conducting training programs. Around 1,25,000 healthcare professionals, including doctors, pharmacists, nurses, drug regulators, patients' support-group and others, had been trained in this regard up to end 2018.

The PvPI has also been integrated with the public health programs such as TB Elimination Program, Universal Immunization Program, Adverse Events Following Immunization, National AIDS Control Organization and National Vector Borne Disease Control Program to identify issues with the safety of medicines and vaccines used in these programs and ensure their safe use. This alignment helps the public health programs to benefit by sharing information on drug alerts and new safety signals generated in respect of drugs/vaccines used in their program.

The inexpensive reporting methods adopted for transmission of information on adverse events (AEs)[6] and ADRs through the PvPI

---

5. Antimicrobial resistance occurs when microorganisms such as bacteria, viruses, fungi and parasites change in ways that render the medications used to cure the infections they cause ineffective. When the microorganisms become resistant to most antimicrobials, they are often referred to as 'superbugs'. (Available at: https://www.who.int/news-room/q-a-detail/antimicrobial-resistance#:~:text=Antimicrobial%20resistance%20occurs%20when%20microorganisms,referred%20to%20as%2)

6. An adverse event refers to an undesirable experience with the use of a medical product. It could include death, hospitalization, disability or permanent damage, congenital anomaly/birth defect or needs intervention to prevent permanent impairment.

structures has improved the ADR reporting scenario in India. It has helped in generating awareness about the effects of new drugs amongst doctors, and alerted them about the possibility of yet unrecognized adverse reactions.

Up to the end of 2019, nearly 0.4 million ADRs data had been assessed by the PvPI, of which 62% were reported by AMCs and public sector (central, states/UTs) teaching hospitals and public health programs and 38% ADRs were reported by the private sector, which includes AMCs and MAHs of pharmaceutical products. Around 71% and 29% of the ADRs reported by public and private sector respectively concerned use of generic medicines. India is, at present, one of the top 10 AD reporting countries in terms of the quality and quantity to WHO-UMC. The National Coordination Centre, PvPI has been recognized by the WHO as one of its Collaborating Centers for Pharmacovigilance in Public Health Programs and Regulatory Services. The WHO has consistently been harping on the point that India needs to play a bigger role in the global landscape of ADR monitoring and become the hub for pharmacovigilance in public health programs and regulatory services.

The PvPI, like all other structures and programs, is not supported by adequate resources and is far from being the ideal structure. The PvPI is currently understaffed. It needs an urgent up gradation and provision of additional resources to enhance its utility.

MATERIOVIGILANCE

The number of adverse events associated with the use of medical technology in healthcare has increased with the passage of time. The risks associated include harmful effects on patients or healthcare professionals; interaction with other substances; contraindications; malfunctioning; technical defects and reduced efficacy of medical devices. The potential risks could sometimes be life threatening and, therefore, it is essential to establish a robust materiovigilance system for identification, collection, reporting and analysis of adverse events associated with the use of medical devices.

Materiovigilance Program of India (MvPI) was launched on July 6, 2015 with the Indian Pharmacopoeia Commission, Ghaziabad as the national coordinating center (NCC). Prior to that, Sree ChitraTirunal Institute of Medical Sciences, Thiruvananthapuram was functioning as the NCC. The program seeks to improve the safety of patients, users and others by reducing the frequency of incidents or adverse events. MvPI is currently working to create a nation-wide system for patient safety monitoring and generating evidence-based data on the safety of medical devices. The program will help in supporting the CDSCO in decision-making in case of medical devices and also for communicating safety information relating to the use of medical devices to various stakeholders to minimize risks. The program also sensitizes manufacturers, importers, distributors of medical devices, including all healthcare stakeholders, for better understanding of medical device standards for promotion of patient safety and strengthening the materiovigilance. It brings both the private and public healthcare delivery system within its fold.

India-specific adverse events reporting tools, technical documents and manuals, training and education kits for stakeholders for reporting ADRs associated with medical devices adverse events have been developed. Though the reporting has increased after the Medical Devices Rules, 2017 came into operation, the MvPI is still at a nascent stage and yet to take firm roots. Unfortunately, for this program also, very limited resources have been provided and the work is being managed largely by the existing PvPI staff.

HAEMOVIGILANCE

The progress in the domain of medical sciences has made it possible to break down blood into different components. The components so fragmented are used for meeting the requirements of different individuals, and the wastage of blood and blood products is minimized. The entire chain – starting with blood donation; its processing and fragmentation into components to the ultimate transfusion in patients – has become a very important aspect of healthcare, especially in some life-threatening diseases.

As in the case of pharmaceuticals and medical devices, the blood transfusion processes need to be monitored to avoid harm to users. The surveillance procedures covering the blood transfusion chain are referred to as Haemovigilance. It involves collection and analysis of data concerning transfusion-related adverse reactions for investigating their causes and outcomes and prevention of their occurrence or recurrence. Transfusion reactions are often not recognized and are under-reported. To ensure uniform practice and safety, every country should have a national haemovigilance system and a set of national guidelines establishing policies for blood transfusion and for detection and management of transfusion reactions.

The Haemovigilance Program of India (HvPI) was launched on 10.12.2012.Over 90 medical colleges across India had been enrolled under the HvPI at the end of 2019. The National Institute of Biologicals (NIB), Noida is the coordinating centre for this program. The NIB has also developed an in-house software 'Haemo-Vigil' for this program. HvPI activities are steered through a core group and an advisory committee for coordinating the haemovigilance activities between medical colleges and the National Coordinating Centre. The committee and the core group also provide expert advice for analysis of information generated. The advisory committee provides insights for linking HvPI with the International Haemo-vigilance Network. The program picked up a lot of momentum during 2015–2018 when the NIB started extensive training for stakeholders from various states. A lot more will need to be done to make the program fully functional.

ADVERSE EVENTS FOLLOWING IMMUNIZATION

A surveillance program to monitor adverse events following immunization (AEFI) has been in operation directly under the MoHFW since 1988. It still suffers from a lack of resources. In 2005, the Government of India had, with the technical assistance from the WHO, drafted the National AEFI Surveillance and Response Operational Guidelines, which were subsequently revised in 2010 and 2015. Many public sector AEFI surveillance workshops have been conducted throughout the country. AEFI surveillance in the private sector is still very limited and needs attention as it also constitutes a critical part of the immunization process.

The CDSCO monitors all post-licensure activities for vaccines, including reported AEFI, periodic safety update reports (PSUR)[7] and any other data on adverse reactions. The CDSCO decisions are based on the analyses of data by an expert committee, recommendations from the National AEFI Committee and investigations, including testing of samples as and when required. As of now, AEFI is loosely structured and the documentation under the program is not up to the mark. It also suffers from the lack of adequate human resources.

SHORTCOMINGS OF THE VIGILANCE MECHANISM

The entire post marketing surveillance system with respect to medical products is still at a nascent stage in India and, therefore, it does not benefit the healthcare system fully. All the four components *viz.* PvPI, MvPI, HvPI and AEFI have been started with minimal resources and still operate with insufficient resources. Given the *ad hoc* nature of manpower engaged in these programs, there are serious question marks on the quality of analysis. Obviously, with *ad hoc* and very meager resources, it can only address routine issues. The outsourced or *ad hoc* manpower might be good for meeting the requirements of data collection and transmission, but better quality of human resources in more numbers will be required for analyzing ADRs, drawing conclusions and making recommendations to the regulatory authorities.

[7.] Periodic Safety Update Report (PSUR) is a document used to provide an update about the safety experience of a medical product to regulatory authorities.

These programs remain restricted to regional ADRs monitoring centers, established at the state/central government-run medical college hospitals and private or corporate hospitals. To reap the full benefit of these programs, the outreach needs to be extended to district and Taluk hospitals and, later, even to primary health centers. The healthcare professionals have not been trained on drug safety and adverse drug reaction reporting. Further, the inability of regulators to initiate and monitor necessary corrective action in a time-bound manner, undermines the efficacy of the entire system.

It is a matter of great concern that adverse interactions of medicines with chemicals, other medicines, food, etc., are often neglected, leading to under- reporting by healthcare professionals as well as patients. It has also been noticed that the private sector has largely been reluctant to participate in the process. This needs to be reversed. There is a general tendency amongst the clinicians, doctors and patients to ignore and not report the adverse reactions to drugs, medical devices and blood transfusion. For the pharmacovigilance system to be efficient, it is important that all stakeholders proactively participate in the process, and that this participation lasts throughout the lifecycle of a medical product.

Non-reporting or gross under-reporting of adverse effects of drugs is on account of a host of reasons including lack of expertise in drug administration. Another major factor contributing for under-reporting is the inadequate nation-wide awareness about the post marketing surveillance. Sometimes the healthcare professionals are reluctant to report adverse events, fearing that this will put them into avoidable legal or other hassles. To counter such reluctance, healthcare professionals need to be assured that submitting a report will not have any legal implications for them.

As of now, only limited data is available for medical device adverse events in India. Engaging consumer societies and organizations for reporting adverse events can be encouraged. Another major handicap of the existing system is that sometimes ADRs are not recognized by physicians at the time of admission. Such unrecognized ADRs could be responsible for the death of many patients or cause serious harm to them.

To sum up, while post marketing surveillance activities (PvPI, MvPI, HvPI and AEFI) are an integral and important part of improving the quality, safety and efficacy of medical products, these activities will need to be suitably stepped up and more resources will need to be committed for undertaking such activities scientifically. At the current level, these activities are not commensurate with the status that the Indian medical products industry wishes to acquire for itself.

CHAPTER 8

DEVELOPMENT OF NEW MEDICAL PRODUCTS

NEED FOR NEWER DRUGS

By now, it is amply clear that medicines play a major role in managing the ever-increasing burden of diseases, both communicable and non-communicable. The lack of preventive healthcare practices, sedentary life style, obsolescence of the existing medicines, newly discovered side effects associated with many existing drugs and antimicrobial resistance arising from the improper use of antibiotics continue to give rise to newer healthcare concerns at regular intervals of time. The changing profile of diseases also throws up unparalleled challenges to health-care providers, researchers and policy makers. The mutation of existing viruses and bacteria, and evolution of altogether new ones continues to confront the system. This makes it imperative to accelerate discovery and development of new drugs.

Quality, safety and efficacy of drugs and the need for strengthening regulatory structures was the focus of the earlier chapters. The present chapter briefly touches upon the processes relating to drug discovery and development, and the role of clinical trials in assessing the quality, safety and efficacy of new drugs. It highlights how clinical trials are important processes associated with drug discovery and development, and that India owing to its vast population and its diversity needs to play a bigger role in the process. It shows that there are serious shortfalls in the translation of basic scientific findings in a laboratory setting to potential treatments for diseases, and that reproducibility and translatability of pre-clinical findings to human applications continues to be a major challenge.

No new efficacious medicines would have been developed without clinical trials, and every medicine or medical device used for treating diverse diseases and conditions or preventing them could be discovered only because someone volunteered to participate in clinical trials, researchers worked systematically to test the safety and efficacy of products and somebody made the necessary resources available for undertaking pre-clinical studies and clinical trials. Development of new drugs or treatment options is both time-consuming and a costly affair. Not undertaking clinical research or conducting clinical trials shuts the door for many new potential treatments. Innovations help in developing new treatment options where there might have been none or provide enhanced efficacy and safety where treatments are already available. As demonstrated by the treatment options used for managing the COVID-19, continued investment in innovations and research & development provides a readymade basis for handling such crisis.

CLINICAL TRIALS

A clinical trial is a systematic study of a new drug or an investigational new drug on human beings for generating data for discovering or verifying its safety, efficacy or tolerance.[1] Clinical trials are preceded by pre-clinical investigations and include animal studies both on non-primates and primates. The safety of drugs in doses equivalent to approximate exposure in human beings is explored through such investigational studies. Any new or investigational drug is permitted to be used in clinical trials only after its safety and efficacy has been ascertained through pre-clinical studies.

Clinical trials are undertaken in four phases. Phase I clinical trials are the first instance in which the new or investigational drug is studied on a small number of healthy volunteers to test the safety and maximum tolerated dose of the drug. Phase II trials are conducted on a small number of volunteers suffering from a disease sought to be treated by using the new or investigational drug. Based on earlier studies, including phase I and phase II clinical trials that demonstrate drug safety and its efficacy, a

---

[1.] Please see New Drugs and Clinical Trial Rules, 2019 notified by the Government of India at: https://cdsco.gov.in/opencms/export/sites/CDSCO_WEB/Pdf-documents/ NewDrugs_ CTRules_2019.pdf

phase III clinical trial is conducted on a larger and more diverse population to demonstrate and confirm the efficacy, and to assess common adverse reactions.

The drugs that fulfill the pre-specified parameters in Phase III trials are approved for marketing in accordance with the conditions of approval. These drugs are subjected to Phase IV trials or post marketing surveillance for identifying longer time adverse reactions that could not have been detected in earlier studies. This phase helps in evaluating the effectiveness of a drug in diseases, populations or doses similar to or markedly different from the original study population and diseases.[2]

The essence of the good clinical research practices is captured in the WHO Handbook on Good Clinical Research Practices.[3] Research involving humans, as per the WHO, needs to be scientifically sound and conducted in accordance with the basic ethical principles that originated from the declaration of Helsinki. It identifies three basic ethical principles, namely respect for persons generally expressed through informed consent; beneficence (the ethical obligation to maximize benefit and to minimize harm); and justice (fair procedures and outcomes in the selection of research subjects), which permeates all other Good Clinical Practices principles (GCP). GCP is an ethical and scientific quality standard for designing, conducting and recording clinical trials that involve participation of human subjects. Compliance with GCP assures the public that the rights, safety and well-being of trial subjects will be protected. It also ensures that clinical trial data are credible.

Improved public health outcomes require a lot more clinical trials to be conducted across different ages, gender and ethnicity of trial subjects. Such trials are also conducted for assessing the merits of a new treatment for people suffering from other health conditions with similar characteristics. The clinical trials assess the benefits, safety or risks of drugs and therapies,

---

[2.] Detailed description of different phases of clinical trials may be seen on Pages 182–184 of the New Drugs and Clinical Trial Rules, 2019 (*ibid*).

[3.] Available on: https://www.who.int/medicines/areas/quality_safety/safety_efficacy/gcp1.pdf

and provide vital information to doctors and patients. They also provide critical insights for improving the existing therapies.

Clinical trials, every time they are conducted, do not necessarily result in the discovery of a blockbuster drug or a medical device, and the success rate in discovery and development of new drugs is very low.

SLOWING DOWN OF NEW DRUG DEVELOPMENT

Owing to a multiplicity of factors, the pool of investible funds available for drug discovery and development has shrunk in the recent past. This poses a serious risk to future human health and well-being. The pace of development of new drugs has also slowed down due to increased pressure on the industry to reduce the cost of drugs in recent times; reduced profit margins of innovator companies, *inter alia*, due to lesser profits as generic medicines are available at a fraction of the cost of branded drugs; and the reduced public investment on research & development in many countries.

As a knowledge-intensive activity, drug discovery and development is a complex process involving a series of activities, starting with the identification of an initial target candidate, pre-clinical studies, clinical trials and ending with post marketing surveillance. Overall, drug discovery and development is a risky and time-consuming process. It requires huge investment in qualified manpower, money, infrastructure and technology. While specific information about the cost of development of new drugs is not available, especially from the private sector, it is assessed that the cost of bringing a prescription drug to the market is in the vicinity of US $ 2–3 billion. The cost of similar development from public-funded institutions is generally lower as a major chunk of expenditure may not get apportioned to a particular study. The cost of drug development is high as of every 8000/10000 new compounds evaluated, only 200/250 reach the animal-testing stage, 5/10 reach human clinical trials stage, out of which one compound only might be approved for human use.

The discovery of a new therapy for a debilitating disease or prevention of epidemics or pandemics provides a ray of hope to millions of human beings. This, coupled with the changing profile of ailments, make it imperative to undertake more clinical research and clinical trials, and create the best possible eco-system for their conduct.

ADHERENCE TO PRESCRIBED PROTOCOLS

Conducting clinical trials, in view of their complexity, requires that the prescribed processes and protocols are followed meticulously. The hazards of not following the protocols could be disastrous, both from the perspective of the harm that might be inflicted on innocent participants as well as legal consequences that could ensue in the light of tightened legal and regulatory requirements across the globe.

Clinical trials related to the human papillomavirus (HPV)[4] with respect to two different vaccines on tribal girls in Andhra Pradesh in 2009 demonstrate the perils of laxity in following the appropriate protocols religiously. In this case, the two HPV vaccines were administered to girls through vaccination camps held at schools and hostels. In a few cases, the consent for vaccination was given by the teacher in charge of a hostel and reportedly by the hostel warden in a few other cases. In a number of cases, the thumb impression had been put. In some cases, the parents of the girls were not told about the vaccination. Many girls who were vaccinated were allegedly pre-pubescent, although the consent form indicated that the vaccine was to be administered to adolescent girls. The matter was all over the media and was also raised in the Indian Parliament repeatedly. It was also examined by the Standing Committee of the Parliament on Health. The issue was also the subject matter of a long drawn-out litigation in the Supreme Court of India.

The case also brought out the darker sides of the clinical trial regime followed in India and highlighted the lapses on the part of the ICMR, the

---

4. Human papillomavirus is a group of over 100 viruses passed through skin-to-skin contact, including through sexual contact. At least, 14 of them are known to be cancer causing. HPV can affect genitals, mouth or throat. HPV vaccines under reference here are used for preventing cervical cancer.

CDSCO, investigators, state government and the vaccine marketers. The lack of adequate regulatory controls had also come up for adverse criticism from the Parliamentary Standing Committee in their 59th and 66th Reports. The media added fuel to the fire by magnifying the shortcomings of the contract research organizations, investigators, medical colleges, the ICMR and other stakeholders. This was despite the fact that in some cases, it was established that the deaths were not related to the administration of vaccines.

The instances of non-adherence with appropriate protocols also led to criticism. The criticism included failure to observe procedural and ethical requirements, bias, problems with documentation, informed consent not having been obtained or obtained inappropriately and some of the incidents, including deaths of clinical trial subjects. The respect for persons, beneficence and justice, the three golden principles enunciated by the WHO and referred to earlier, had been completely ignored in most of the clinical trials conducted in India. This resulted in a massive campaign against the conduct of clinical trials.

Notwithstanding the above, introducing newer and more efficacious medicines for handling the growing disease burden is indispensable in the context of the changing profile of diseases. The alternative of abandoning clinical research and clinical trials is not acceptable. While observing due diligence, these activities have to continue in the larger interest of the humanity. This is especially so in view of the complexity involved in developing newer drugs as well as the potency of such drugs. Following the best regulatory practices for complying with the requirements of quality, safety and efficacy of such products and related bioethical concerns is, therefore, critical. Safeguarding the interests of participants in clinical trials by minimizing the risks associated with them and ensuring the safety of clinical trial participants by keeping the required mitigation measures handy, is also an important consideration.

Democratic polity, freedom of speech and expression bordering a license to say what one pleases and free media that are excessively obsessed with TRP sometimes turn out to be a deadly cocktail. It inhibits decision making or results in decisions being made in such a manner that cater to the popular sentiments rather than be based on rationality, reason and science. The story of clinical trials in India, post the HPV clinical trials in Andhra Pradesh referred to earlier, manifests this aspect very clearly.

SCALE AND SCOPE OF CLINICAL TRIALS

Notwithstanding the shrinking budgets, with the need for newer medicines becoming more pronounced by the day, rough estimates are that the scale of the global clinical trials industry would be in the vicinity of US $ 90 billion by 2030, with a compound annual growth rate of over 6%. The chronic diseases and conditions, and the new emerging threats, such as pandemics, will be the main drivers of clinical trials in future.

Till now, the clinical trial market has primarily been dominated by the USA. The large and diverse pool of patients and the prevalence of diseases and health conditions in India provide a good base for the clinical trial industry in the country. After the agreement on Trade Related aspects of Intellectual Property in 2005, there was a significant increase in the number of clinical trials in India. The increase in the number of clinical trials after 2005 created newer employment opportunities and led to the emergence of a new class of entrepreneurs to run clinical research organizations, and bioavailability and bioequivalence centers. The success of the clinical trial industry, however, proved to be short-lived owing to the inadequate regulatory safeguards that resulted in a number of complications during 2010–2013. A number of cases of alleged trial data falsification, lack of informed consent and inadequate compensation also came to light.

The Public Interest Litigation by a non-governmental organization 'Swasthya Adhikar Manch' in the Supreme Court relating to HPV vaccine referred to earlier, cajoled the government out of slumber. In a knee-jerk reaction, a lot of restrictions were imposed without detailed analysis of the pros & cons to curb the malpractices noticed in the conduct of clinical trials. The remedy turned out to be the nemesis of the clinical trial industry in the country, and the conduct of clinical trials in India came to a grinding halt. Unfortunately, even at that point of time, the strengthening of regulatory structures for better oversight of clinical trials got sidestepped.

INDIA'S POTENTIAL IN THE CLINICAL TRIAL INDUSTRY

The large and diverse patient pool with variations in terms of ethnicity and disease patterns; skilled human resources comprising scientists, clinicians; a pharmaceutical industry on the upswing; medical colleges and institutes; clinical trial sites, other related institutions in the country and the prowess in the field of information technology – all of these factors augur well for establishing a robust ecosystem for the conduct of clinical trials in India. Currently, with over 17% of the world population and nearly one-fifth of the global disease burden, India has the potential to be one of the top destinations for conducting clinical trials and new drug discovery and development.

It would not be an exaggeration to say that many public institutions in India are capable of contributing significantly in the process of development of new drugs and therapies. It is another matter that their potential has not been harnessed. India's indigenous, inactivated vaccine against COVID-19, COVAXIN, manufactured by Bharat Biotech and developed in collaboration with the National Institute of Virology, ICMR with inputs from the Indian Institute of Chemical Technology (IICT), CSIR is a pointer to the high potential of collaboration between the public and the private sector for exploring new frontiers. This, however, is one odd example of successful leveraging of the strengths of the private and the public sector. There are many more examples to the contrary.

The scope for collaboration between publicly funded institutes and industry on innovation-focused research initiatives is huge. Rather than working in silos, there is a need for evolving a collaborative approach and harness this potential for establishing the credentials of the country in drug discovery and development. A number of scientific institutions in the public sector are working on the same or related areas, but they continue to work independently without sharing resources or information with each other.

Some developments in the recent past could help in furthering conversion of the basic scientific research into actual deliverables. Setting up of the Translational Health Science and Technology Institute (THSTI), a part of the inter-disciplinary Biotech Science Cluster at Faridabad, National Capital Region, is one such positive development. It has been designed as an interactive organization with a mission to conduct innovative translational research across disciplines and professions to accelerate development of concepts into products to improve human health. The Bangalore Life Sciences Cluster is another effort aimed at establishing some degree of synergy in research. Many more collaborations of this nature, and also with the private sector would be required to steer the research to the next level by optimal utilization of available resources.

ABSENCE OF CLEAR REGULATIONS FOR CLINICAL TRIALS

As stated earlier, clinical trials need to be conducted in accordance with the protocols and regulations that have been evolved in the form of national laws and rules, and international best practices, standards, procedures, guidance documents, etc., to ensure that the new therapies and drugs are safe and effective, and the potential risks of untested drugs to human beings are minimized. The absence of clear clinical trial rules and practices and non-compliance with global good practices in India has been a major dampener.

Clinical trials in India were earlier conducted in accordance with the Drugs & Cosmetics Rules, 1945. However, as these did not contain specific provisions on a number of issues, such trials were guided by a patchwork of rules and non-binding international ethical standards and practices. Besides being unpredictable, this vested the authorities concerned with widespread discretion with no clear guidance to address many facets of clinical trials.

In the aftermath of the Public Interest Litigation in the Supreme Court of India in 2012 referred to earlier, alleging malpractices in the conduct of clinical trials, both by governmental and non-governmental organizations and also by independent investigators, the apex court opined that approvals for clinical trials should be based on all relevant aspects of safety and efficacy, particularly with regard to the assessment of risk versus benefit to the patients, innovation *vis-à-vis* existing therapeutic options and unmet medical needs in the country.

The tightening of the clinical trials regime led to a steep drop in the number of clinical trials conducted in the country between 2010 (500 trials) and 2013 (19 trials). This delayed introduction of new medicines in the country.

Before framing of the New Drugs & Clinical Trials Rules, 2019, clinical trials in India were regulated by the provisions of Rules 122A, 122 B, 122C, 122D, 122DA, 122DAA and 122E and Schedule 'Y' of the Drugs and Cosmetics Rules, 1945. After observations of the Supreme Court, a number of amendments were carried out in these Rules in October 2013.

Newly introduced Rule 122DAB, *inter alia*, provided for financial compensation over and above free medical management to an affected clinical trial participant in case of injury or death during clinical trials. The authority for determining the quantum of compensation was vested in the Central Licensing Authority. Another rule, *viz.* 122DAC, *inter alia*, introduced the requirement to comply with Schedule Y of the Drugs & Cosmetics Rules, 1945 and obtaining approval of an Ethics Committee; registration of the clinical trials with the Clinical Trials Registry of India; submission of reports of serious adverse events, etc.

The procedure for regulating clinical trials evolved over a period of time and has been amended several times in an *ad hoc* manner. As a result of frequent changes, some of the issues lacked clarity and many provisions were also not consistent with international practices. Most of the countries, including the USA, had been highlighting problems with the rules and regulatory practices relating to conduct of clinical trials in India. The major concerns expressed by the clinical trial industry in India and abroad were the lack of transparency and unpredictability in the disposal of applications for conducting clinical trials; inadequacy of regulatory structures, both in terms of knowledge and capacity, to deal with the quantum of work resulting in undue delay in the disposal of applications; repeated queries by the committees; and concerns regarding patient safety and compensation to be provided to participants in the event of any adverse effects suffered by them.

After the intervention of the Supreme Court, the proposals seeking approval for conduct of clinical trials had to be placed before a three-tiered structure comprising the Subject Expert Committee; the Technical Committee headed by DGHS; and the Apex Committee headed by Secretary, MoHFW. The meetings of these committees were irregular and, very often, the decisions lacked scientific basis. While the Technical Committee often raised a number of queries, there was hardly any value addition by the Apex Committee. It only entailed additional paper work and wastage of time in finding answers to the queries, many of which were scientifically not relevant.

IMPROVING THE CLINCAL TRIAL ENVIRONMENT

During 2014–17, a lot of efforts were made to improve the regulatory practices including those concerning clinical trials in the country and make the processes transparent and time bound so that clinical trials could start again and the Indian population was not made to wait for new medicines. During this time, the Indian GCP guidelines were formulated by an Expert Committee set up by the CDSCO. These provided for uniform quality of clinical research throughout the country and generated data for registration of new drugs before use in the Indian population.

As per the GCP, a clinical trial applicant was required to submit an application to the CDSCO along with full product details; animal pharmacology and toxicity data; animal toxicology and clinical data, if available; the trial protocol; and information about the regulatory status of the product in other countries. Applicants also had to report any suspected or unexpected serious adverse reaction of the product in other countries.

Institutional ethics committees (IECs) were asked to review and monitor clinical trials for compliance with ethical guidelines.[5] Additional requirements were introduced for the informed consent process and mandatory audio-visual recording to protect vulnerable subjects in line with international best practices. From 2011, registration of ethics committees with the licensing authority had also been made mandatory.

The Handbook on clinical trial applications was also published in January 2017, and the training of Subject Expert Committee members and the CDSCO reviewers was stepped up. Timelines for review of clinical trial applications were reduced by increasing the number of members on Subject Expert panels and an online submission process was started for approval of clinical trial applications. Timelines for serious adverse event reporting by investigators, ethics committees and sponsors were also rationalized. For clinical trials of recombinant DNA-derived products, a parallel submission process to Review by the Committee on Genetic Manipulation (RCGM) and the CDSCO was introduced to cut down the delay in the process. However, these were all stop-gap arrangements and there was a need for evolving a coherent legal framework for clinical trials.

Prof. Ranjit Roy Chaudhury, a key adviser to the then Health and Family Welfare Ministry, did a commendable work for institutionalizing the payment of compensation in the event of injury or death of a clinical trial participant. The then Additional Secretary in the MoHFW, R.K. Jain, steered the entire process and also helped develop an objective criteria for handling issues relating to payment of compensation and commencing the work for fine-tuning other aspects of clinical trials.

WORK ON NEW DRUGS AND CLINICAL TRIAL RULES

Detailed discussions with different associations of industry as well as consumers and other stakeholders on matters relating to regulation of clinical trials were organized at the level of Joint Secretary, MoHFW during 2015-17.

[5.] IECs review safety reports, informed consent document and violations of ethical guidelines.

These helped in forging consensus on the basis of best international practices for conduct and regulation of clinical trials in the country. The process of drafting new rules for regulating new drugs and clinical trials in the country was kick-started in the right earnest, and all relevant information for the same was collected from different sources. Many stakeholders, including the Indian Society for Clinical Research (ISCR), contributed towards fostering an understanding of the clinical trial-related matters.

While the work relating to drafting of new rules was still in progress, in a meeting of the Apex Committee set up for monitoring the progress of clinical trials, the then Secretary, Department of Health Research highlighted that in the absence of any law, the Department was finding it difficult to regulate certain aspects concerning biomedical and health research. It was indicated that the enactment of a new law was also nowhere on the horizon. It was agreed that as an interim arrangement, a provision for this may be added in the New Drug & Clinical Trial Rules that was being drafted by MoHFW.

With the help of a small cell of six persons, including three attending to Hindi translation of other rules, the draft of the new rules for clinical trial-related matters was ready for being referred to the Legislative Department for vetting in the third week of May 2017. Going beyond the normal call of their official duties, a large number of officials from the CDSCO participated in the discussions every weekend and almost every other day after office hours. However, the process of vetting got delayed due to senior officers of MoHFW being busy in the meeting of the World Health Assembly in Geneva.

With the change of the incumbent Joint Secretary in June 2017, for nearly a year there was no major progress in the matter. Under pressure from the Supreme Court, the matter had to be reconsidered and after vetting by the Legislative Department, the draft rules were published in the *Gazette of India* on 01.02.2018, i.e., nearly eight months after these rules were ready for soliciting comments of stakeholders.

After the matter was taken up in the Supreme Court in December 2018 and the government had to give a commitment, the rules were eventually notified on 19.03. 2019. No doubt, finalizing the rules was an arduous task, especially as it had to be done without any additional manpower. The fact that it took all the time from May 2017 to March 2019 to notify the rules, the draft of which was already there, indicates the low priority accorded to the work. It is also important to note that it took so long despite the intervention of the Supreme Court.

NEW DRUGS AND CLINICAL TRIAL RULES

The New Drugs and Clinical Trial Rules, 2019 replaced Part XA and Schedule Y of the Drugs & Cosmetics Rules, 1945, which was a conglomeration of many piecemeal efforts made over a period of time. The new rules are applicable to, and regulate all new drugs, investigational new drugs for human use, clinical trials, bioequivalence studies, bioavailability studies and Ethics Committees, etc.

The rules clearly define new drugs, investigational new drugs, orphan drugs, academic clinical trials and other related terms. It reduces the chances of any misinterpretation. The rules also bring a high degree of clarity regarding definition of various terms and the constitution, role and scope of the work entrusted to the Ethics Committees, both for clinical trials, and biomedical and health research. The rules also specify the timelines for clearance or rejection of various types of proposals by the Central Licensing Authority and the concept of deemed approval has been introduced. As per the provisions of these rules, in the event of non-adherence with timelines, the clearances will be deemed to have been granted.

The new rules provide that no clearance is required from the Central Licensing Authority for conduct of academic clinical trials. The requirement of local clinical trials has been dispensed with in case of drugs approved in well-regulated countries. The clinical trial participants are now entitled to get post- trial access to investigational new drugs. Medical management will now be required to be provided to clinical trial participants as long as required in the opinion of the investigator or till such time it is not established that the injury is not related to the clinical trials.

The major adverse events associated with clinical trials are death, development of an adverse reaction, relapse and the onset of a new disease. Provisions have since been made in the new rules for providing compensation to clinical trial participants in the event of any of these happening. The requirements of animal toxicology studies, teratogenic studies,[6] peri-natal studies, mutagenicity[7] and carcinogenicity studies have been relaxed in case of new drugs that have been approved and marketed for more than two years in identified countries.

The definition of the new drugs in these rules is of special significance. A new drug includes, *inter alia*, active pharmaceutical ingredient or phyto-pharmaceutical drug, which has not been used in the country to any significant extent; a drug approved by the Central Licensing Authority for certain claims and proposed to be marketed with modified or new claims; a fixed dose combination of two or more drugs, approved separately for certain claims and proposed to be combined for the first time in a fixed ratio; a modified or sustained release form of a drug or novel drug delivery system of any drug approved by the Central Licensing Authority; or a vaccine, recombinant Deoxyribonucleic Acid (r-DNA) derived product; living modified organism; monoclonal anti-body; stem cell derived product; gene therapeutic product or xenografts,[8] intended to be used as a drug.

The new rules lay out a predictable, transparent and objective framework for ethical conduct of clinical trials in India. This has restored the confidence of the clinical trial industry to a large extent, and it will lead to faster approvals and availability of new drugs in India. In the absence of updated Drugs & Cosmetics law that remained pending for years, these rules bring in much desired clarity about the regulatory requirements for conducting clinical trials in India.

[6.] Teratology is the science of studying and investigating birth defects and their etiologies.

[7.] Mutagenicity refers to the mutation or change in the DNA of a cell. The changes in DNA as a consequence of mutagens could harm cells and cause certain diseases. Radioactive substances, X-rays, ultraviolet radiation and some chemicals are mutagens.

[8] Xenografts are tissue grafts or organ transplant from a donor of a species other than the recipient.

The absence of an updated parliamentary law might have led to some overstepping beyond the existing legislative framework. However, the rules could perhaps not have done any better. There are a few issues that could possibly be construed to be going beyond the scope of the parent legislation, though not eroding the spirit of the Act. The two such areas are the provisions relating to Ethics Committee for biomedical research and the mechanism evolved for awarding compensation to trial subjects in cases of death or injury. There are still many areas that need to be addressed.

ENHANCING TRANSPARENCY

The lack of transparency in clinical research and clinical trials gives rise to suspicions due to suppression of the details relating to studies, design of such studies and trials and the negative outcomes.[9] This also hinders clinical research and leads to avoidable expenditure on many facets that would have been covered by previous studies. It would serve the cause of public health better if a system could be evolved for sharing the information regarding clinical research and trials by placing all pertinent details in the public domain from where these could be easily retrieved, accessed and used for future research.

The information should, *inter alia*, contain details of successful, unsuccessful and discontinued trials and any other details that could foster future clinical research. This might entail evolving some compensation mechanism for those who share such details. In any case, where R&D has been conducted using public money, the details should mandatorily be placed in the public domain. It would help in expanding the frontiers of scientific knowledge, reduce costs associated with conducting clinical research and trials and using such knowledge for ensuring better healthcare to many more.

Some beginning to bring in higher transparency in this regard has already been made and the Draft Technology, and Innovation Policy of

---

[9.] This is one of the major criticisms of the pharmaceutical industry. For details see Chapter 1.

the Government of India released in December 2020[10] has proposed to establish an all-encompassing Open Science Framework to provide access to scientific data, information, knowledge and resources to everyone in the country. Accordingly, all data used in and generated from publicly funded research will be available to everyone under findable, accessible, interoperable and reusable (FAIR) terms.

PUBLIC FUNDING FOR DRUGS WITH LOWER RETURN

There is a serious incoherence between market-driven research and public health. The market-driven research & development mostly focuses on areas that have huge markets. New technologies are rarely developed to address diseases that do not yield high returns. Orphan drugs are a case in point. Some way needs to be found for addressing this issue. It is also now critical to break the microbial resistance cycle and make a major investment in new antimicrobial drugs and to control their use to ensure that they also do not succumb to antimicrobial resistance.

TRANSLATIONAL SERVICES

The basic research in natural sciences can lead to discoveries that could help improve human health. However, moving the discoveries from bench to bedside through clinical trials still remains a major challenge. The translational gap is particularly prominent in the pharmaceutical industry. Despite many scientific advances, the development of innovative drugs has continued to decline with a high rate of failure in clinical trials. The predictive capabilities of the technologies, such as artificial intelligence (AI), can be leveraged to streamline clinical research and clinical trial processes, and select the right study design. AI can also be used to replace a large number of manual processes. Successful leveraging of the artificial intelligence and machine learning can also shorten the clinical research and clinical trial pathways.

---

10. Available on https://dst.gov.in/sites/default/files/STIP Doc_1.4_Dec2020.pdf

MISSING ECOSYSTEM FOR CLINICAL RESEARCH

The availability of scientific and technical manpower notwithstanding, clinical research in India is not that well-structured. As of now, the clinical research in India is confined to a narrow base and in many cases, the Indian industry prefers the research to be undertaken abroad owing to a host of factors, including delay in approvals and excessive restrictions on the use of animals in the process of clinical research for establishing the safety and efficacy of the potential drugs. In such circumstances, it becomes easier for the innovators to undertake research, including animal toxicological studies, in foreign universities or establishments. Owing to restrictions on conducting pre-clinical studies on animals, especially on primates, most Indian companies prefer to conduct such studies outside India.

Clinical trials involve a rigorous approach on the basis of scientific, statistical, ethical and legal considerations. Unfortunately, a large number of personnel working in the area of clinical trial or clinical research are not familiar with the ethical and other requirements. It is, therefore, crucial for healthcare providers to understand the clinical trials processes for maintaining a partnership with patients and industry in pursuit of the safest, most effective and efficient therapies. Addressing the acute shortage of qualified human resources for effectively handling clinical research and clinical trials would need introduction of appropriate courses in Indian universities in partnership with the existing structures in the public sector. Such human resources should also be proficient in the use of information technology, artificial intelligence and machine learning tools for optimal utilization of resources.

HARMONIZATION OF PRACTICES

Since clinical trials are conducted globally, it is necessary that a uniform set of processes, procedures and practices are adopted everywhere for conducting clinical trials. It will be necessary to take the work of harmonization of the global practices forward and make globally acceptable mandatory standards/regulations for governing clinical research/trials. Ensuring the safety of participants in the clinical trials as well as preserving the integrity and credibility of the data reported, stringent regulatory structures comprising competent and qualified personnel are required to be established. Findings of the actual clinical practice will need to complement the validity established on the basis of narrowly selective enrollment criteria and artificial setting within which a clinical trial is conducted.

To conclude, it can be said that clinical trials and clinical research have continued to be neglected in India. Despite availability of scientific and technical manpower, clinical trials and clinical research are still not that well-structured. As of now, clinical research in India is confined to a narrow base. There is also an acute shortage of qualified human resources for effectively undertaking clinical research and clinical trials. A nurturing ecosystem for conducting clinical research and trials is missing and the institutional mechanisms for approval, monitoring and conduct of clinical trials is highly restrictive. Adopting and integrating interdisciplinary approach through the use of technologies, such as artificial intelligence and machine learning, would help in making the outcomes predictable, reduce errors in data analysis and also reduce costs.

Many public institutions in India are capable of contributing significantly towards the process of development of new drugs and therapies. India could be at the forefront of clinical research and clinical trials, and thus help in furthering the cause of the humanity to a large extent by leveraging the demographic dividend and generating employment in the cutting edge research. However, for this, it would be necessary to create the right ecosystem in terms of infrastructure, well-trained researchers, better laboratory facilities, clear and predictable processes to handle all research-related activities. Further, adherence with the good medical records/ documentation practices; introduction of quality control system that can identify and resolve issues in time; robust consent process; timely and complete adverse events reporting; subject safety management; adequate subject protection and predictable and stringent regulatory framework will be necessary. The direction for all this has to come from the government.

CHAPTER 9

DOMESTIC MANUFACTURING OF QUALITY DRUGS, INCLUDING API

The enactment of the Indian Patents Act, 1970 paved the way for the fast-paced growth of the Indian pharmaceutical industry. This could, however, not be supplemented by an appropriate ecosystem for providing a clear direction to the industry through suitable incentives and disincentives. Along with the sub-optimal regulation and the weak institutions that did not have the required resources or governmental support, these factors complete the story about the neglect of the pharmaceutical sector. The lack of ownership and abandonment of the sector led to the chaotic growth of the Indian pharmaceuticals industry and also confined its scope to low-cost generics. The generic medicines of Indian origin have not been without controversy, and this book has provided details of that in ample measure in previous chapters.

The excessive dependence on raw material alleged to be of inferior quality, sourced largely from China has, along with a few other factors discussed earlier, led to the manufacturing of relatively poor-quality formulations in India. That the neglect relates to the pharmaceutical sector which has enjoyed a consistent and long run 'Revealed Comparative Advantage' in exports since 2009,[1] speaks volumes about the mismanagement of the sector.

The present chapter focuses on redeeming the stature of the Indian pharmaceutical industry through reduced imports, moving beyond generics and making India the *bona fide* pharmacy of the world. It highlights that the quality of medical products, nurturing environment for the industry

[1] *Economic Survey 2020–21*, Government of India, page 97–98, Volume 2.

and investment in research & development, especially in the innovation space, could only steer the future growth of the Indian pharmaceutical industry.

THREAT TO THE INDIAN GENERIC INDUSTRY

The Indian pharmaceutical sector is predominantly engaged in manufacturing low-cost generic drugs for meeting the domestic demand as well as exports. As compared with 1991 when India was importing only 0.3% of its Active Pharmaceutical Ingredients (API)/Key Starting materials (KSM)/Drug Intermediate (DI) from China, in 2021, over 70% of the pharmaceutical industry requirement for the raw material is being met by imports from China. At this rate, any disruption of supplies from China can bring the so-called pharmacy of the world to a grinding halt, especially as there are no alternatives for procuring API in such large quantities. The Indian formulation industry is today at crossroads for a variety of reasons. The fragilities associated with the supply chain of low-cost API/ KSM/DI have suddenly increased in the backdrop of the changing geo-strategic environment post the onset of the COVID-19 pandemic; India's association with the quad comprising Australia, India, Japan and the USA; the hostilities on Indo-China Line of Actual Control; and the US–China trade war. The tightening of environmental controls in China in the recent past has also not made the situation any better as far as supply of API to the Indian industry is concerned.

China is also entering the formulation business and, given its ability to scale things up, it does not portend well for the Indian generic industry. China has made concerted efforts to strengthen its national drug regulatory structures in the recent past, and harmonization with global practices is being attempted in a big way. China has also decided to join PIC/S.[2] India has, in comparison, been content with the dysfunctional

---

[2.] The Pharmaceutical Inspection Co-operation Scheme (PIC/S) is an informal, co-operative and non-binding arrangement between Medical Products Regulatory Authorities that have comparable Good Manufacturing Practices for medical products for human or veterinary use.

regulatory structures, as highlighted in the earlier chapters, and very little effort has been made to harmonize with global best practices. There is still no concerted move to join PIC/S. Another aspect that cannot be ignored is that no country, not even India, can think of creating global multinational companies without proper direction from the government and its active support to make such companies globally competitive. This will entail the evolution of a calibrated policy and its meticulous execution.

A number of new players in South Asia, East Asia, Africa, Latin America and Eastern Europe are entering the formulations market. The competition from Brazil, Indonesia, Bangladesh, Sri Lanka, Turkey, Egypt, Jordan, China, Morocco, Tunisia and Ethiopia, etc., will be formidable in the near future. It could be a potential threat to the Indian formulation industry in the longer run. This is especially so as some of the concerns relating to the quality of Indian medicines are for real and it might not be difficult for the new players to supply medicines of comparable quality even at a cost lower than that of the Indian generics.

With plenty of cheap labor and a number of factories, making generic drugs is no big deal. It is the quality of the product that can make Indian generics useful and marketable. The time is not far off when medicines could be manufactured in fully automated factories with minimal human intervention. If the quality is lacking, cheap labor or the so-called demographic dividend alone can work no longer.

Another important aspect that needs to be taken into account is that many countries are concerned about the lack of alternative sources for supply of medicines as they consider dependence on a single source problematic. Countries such as the USA are already contemplating diversifying the sourcing of generic medicines.

In the emerging global scenario, India does not have a choice in so far as strengthening of the domestic manufacturing of drugs, including API, is concerned. The constraints, both on account of availability of API/KSM/DI for the reasons stated above and the demand for formulations due to quality concerns, could adversely affect the Indian economy as a whole in view of the current size and the reach of India's pharmaceutical industry.

QUALITY API FOR QUALITY FORMULATIONS

Medicines cure diseases, but they could also be very harmful if their quality is compromised. During synthesis of API, many unwanted chemicals called impurities are also produced. Such impurities have no clinical value but have the potential to harm the patient. Sometimes, impurities associated with raw materials find their way into the API when they escape the purification process as their properties resemble the main compound.[3] Detecting and removing all impurities in API is not always possible. In the event of their non-removal, the impurities impact the quality of formulations adversely. The Heparin disaster of 2008 was a consequence of quality compromises in API supplied by China and is a grim reminder of how dangerous such quality compromises could be.

For the benefit of discerning readers, Heparin is a natural product found in pig's blood vessels. It is refined and made into an API. In the 2008 disaster, 81 people died as heparin, a blood thinner used in surgeries and dialysis, made from Chinese API had serious quality issues. Baxter, the pharmaceutical company, used the API Heparin imported from China to make finished dosages and released heparin injections and solutions for marketing in the US market. The medication caused serious adverse reactions such as allergy and low blood pressure in patients and also resulted in deaths, as stated above.

During investigation, the US FDA found that Heparin API was contaminated with over-sulfated chondroitin sulfate. Further investigation revealed that due to the shortage of the required type of pigs and cost considerations, the Chinese manufacturers of Heparin chose an alternative route to meet the requirements. They used Chondroitin sulfate which is also a natural product and is made from animal cartilage but is cheaper than crude Heparin and mimics real Heparin. The Chinese manufacturer of Heparin adulterated the API with over-sulfated chondroitin sulfate which could not be identified during routine laboratory tests.

[3.] https://www.pharmatimesnow.com/2018/11/5-things-about-active-pharmaceutical-ingredients.html

In the Indian milieu, the concerns are more serious in view of the fact that the chances of filtering the inferior quality API are negligible, given the weak regulatory structures. In this context, it is worth noting that the inspectors of the CDSCO who had inspected API manufacturing sites in China had pointed out that the API was lying in the open on the roads. However, after those findings, no further inspections of API manufacturing sites in China could be undertaken.

In 2016, inspections of API manufacturers in China were proposed to be resumed and a roster of inspectors and other senior drug regulatory officials was prepared for it. When the file was put up for approval, the then Additional Secretary put it in a spin and the proposal never materialized. As a result, the inspections of Chinese API facilities could not be undertaken and the API of suspect quality continues to be imported in large quantities for making formulations. The import of inferior quality API has also continued to be highlighted in the media; however, for a long period, no concrete remedial actions have been taken. It needs to be clearly understood that quality formulations require quality raw materials and quality API/KSM/DI. Their poor quality can produce only poor quality formulations.

MISPLACED VISION AND MUDDLED DIRECTION

Goals, milestones and strategic direction should ideally flow from a clear vision. If the vision is vague and the activities are directionless, the outcomes are bound to be sub-optimal. On the other hand, in spite of the existence of a clear vision, if the direction and ownership of the top management is missing, the goals cannot be achieved. Unfortunate as it is, the Indian medical products industry suffers the twin disadvantages: the vision is hazy and there is no ownership either by the political leadership or senior echelons of bureaucracy.

India's overwhelming dependence on China for API reflects poorly on the vision of India's policy makers. It exhibits that the political executive and the senior bureaucracy that was supposed to render its services in an apolitical manner for the efficient transformation of the economy and the society in the post-independence era, failed the country. The liberalized regime, post 1991, in general, and after 2005 in particular, facilitated import-driven growth of the pharmaceutical sector and also helped in the decimation of India's API industry. We also need to take note of the fact that in 1977–78, many Indian industries were at least 10 years ahead of China in producing API. In 2021, the best Indian companies are at least 10 years behind China in the same area.

The concerns relating to the quality of API sourced for manufacturing formulations have been in the knowledge of the Indian authorities for decades, and so has the fact that with poor quality API, it is difficult to produce quality formulations. In order to address concerns in this regard, a number of studies have been undertaken in the past. These also examined the aspects relating to boosting the domestic manufacturing of API and reduce import dependence. The findings and recommendations of such studies have remained on paper, barring the occasional but inadequate governmental response. One of the problematic areas has also been the lukewarm participation of industry in such studies, with the result that these produced reports that contained only the perspective of government officials, who despite their diligence had little knowledge about running business.

The lack of production of bulk drugs[4] in adequate quantities in the country had also figured prominently in the report of the Hathi Committee submitted as early as in 1975. It had found that only 64 units in the organized sector were producing bulk drugs. The report had highlighted that most of the production was from the penultimate stage and largely for captive consumption. It also pointed out that there was very little enthusiasm for manufacturing bulk drugs from raw materials. In 1973, the value of bulk drug production in India was only to the tune of Rs. 240 crore, of which one-third was produced by PSUs. The position has only deteriorated after that.

The danger of depending excessively on the Chinese API continued to be highlighted even after that from time to time. In 2013, a committee

---

4. The term bulk drugs and API are used interchangeably in this book.

headed by Dr. V.M. Katoch (the then Secretary, Health Research and Director General, Indian Council of Medical Research) was set up to examine the concerns on this issue. The committee had, in its report submitted in 2015, proposed several measures. These included setting up of six large clusters/large manufacturing zones/parks for API, single window clearance, common facilities such as effluent treatment plant, testing facilities/laboratories, assistance for IPR management, design, etc., providing capex loan/interest subvention, zero duties/taxes and concessional and timely allocation of coal and uninterrupted power supply to boost domestic production of APIs. The list of incentives to be provided was comprehensive; however, it could not be taken to a logical conclusion.[5] While it needs to be admitted that this report could perhaps not have been implemented in totality, it could have been the beginning for evolving a clear direction for the sector through the involvement of the stakeholders.

DECIMATION OF THE INDIAN API INDUSTRY

Free trade is, no doubt, important for the creation of wealth, economic development and prosperity across countries. It should, however, not be allowed to create monopolies and cartels. The imperfections of the market need to be duly taken note of while pursuing free trade. No country will prefer to remain the supplier of only the raw material and leave other countries to do the value addition. Indian policy makers, through their actions and omissions, blunted the opportunity for the Indian pharmaceutical industry to become the largest supplier of API/KSM. As a result, the Chinese API/KSM became the mainstay of the Indian pharmaceutical industry and now China, with the help of Indian professionals, is seeking to leverage the expertise in API manufacturing for production of formulations.

The price controls through National Pharmaceuticals Pricing Authority also forced the manufacturers to shift to the imported cheaper

---

[5] Salient features of Katoch Committee recommendations are available at: https://pharmaceuticals.gov.in/sites/default/files/Katoch%20Committe%20Report_0.pdf

but inferior quality API for manufacturing formulations. The pressure to reduce the prices of formulations led the manufacturers to scout for cheaper alternatives of raw materials, and there was none other than China where the scale and the substantial government subsidy and incentives helped reduce the costs. As a consequence, with reduced demand and no governmental support, the Indian API industry became unviable. What is worse is that the price controls were also applied to the API.

Indian Drugs and Pharmaceutical Limited and Hindustan Antibiotics Limited manufactured several lifesaving drugs like penicillin, streptomycin and sulpha-drugs, and made them available at affordable prices.[6] However, suitable policy interventions were not initiated for decades and the imperfections of market tilted the scales in favor of China. The decline and fall of the public sector pharmaceutical companies over a period of time was the result of the gross neglect of the sector by administrative departments, the lack of vision of the political leadership; inability of the bureaucracy to act in the national interest; and more than anything else, starving of these units by denying them adequate resources.

The loss of the public sector to a large extent was partially to the benefit of the private sector, which prospered. However, most of the units in the private sector focused only on areas that fetched short-term higher returns and, of course, it was not manufacturing API for various reasons alluded to above.

Another major factor that constrained the development of capacity for manufacturing bulk drugs was the license-permit Raj. Today, for the younger generations, it would be difficult to visualize how the entrepreneurs in different sectors must have dealt with the overbearing bureaucracy during the first four/five decades of India's independence. An officer who had worked as Deputy Controller of Capital Issues in the Department of Economic Affairs in 1980s once stated that the doyens of Indian industry had to wait for hours before being able to meet him. That was just a sample of the unrestrained power that the bureaucracy wielded

---

6. Reddy, K. Anji: *An Unfinished Agenda* (Page 18–19).

in India. The officials working in the departments dealing with issuance of licenses exercised authority with an iron fist. The unfettered discretion that they possessed during license-permit Raj was unparalleled. It stifled the Indian initiative to a large extent in the same manner as non-pragmatic environmental conditions on animal studies and others are constraining research and development at present.

The governmental machinery during the license-permit Raj and even later, was least interested in creating an environment conducive for voluntarily taking up the manufacturing of bulk drugs through appropriate incentives. In fact, any facilitation of industrial development or developing efficient manufacturing processes and introducing measures for quality management in production did not form part of the public discourse at that point of time and even much later. On the contrary, some degree of coercion was deployed by the government to force manufacturers to take up bulk drugs production.

In contrast to India, the emergence of China as a major supplier of API was facilitated by the economies of scale and aggressive governmental support in terms of capex, subsidized interest on loans, free land, electricity and water, and that resulted in lowering the cost of API by over 40%. China incentivized its industry to undercut competition to the disadvantage of the Indian industry.

The Indian pharmaceutical companies preferred importing API from China to manufacturing it in-house or procuring from domestic sources as the latter was a costly affair. In the absence of any major support coming from the government, the API manufacturing was largely abandoned by the Indian industry, and only selective and captive facilities were retained for a miniscule number of products.

NEGLECT OF THE PUBLIC SECTOR VACCINE MANUFACTURERS

The story of institutions set up to manufacture vaccines in the public sector is no different. The neglect of institutions such as the Central Research Institute (CRI), Kasauli, Pasteur Institute of India, Coonoor, the BCG

Vaccine Laboratory, Chennai and HLL Biotech Ltd. (HBL), a recent state-of-the-art WHO-pre-qualified facility at Chengalpattu, Chennai reflects the mismanagement by the government. Currently, all these institutions do not have the required resources and most of their time, money and energy is wasted in seeking approvals from the arrogant governmental structures. In the process, these have, despite good infrastructure, become national liabilities. It is time to redefine the roles of such institutions and make them fully autonomous and self-sustaining. Their activities need to be stepped up so that they can contribute in furtherance of good healthcare in the country. Eventually, they must move out of the government's control. Permitting excellent state-of-the art facilities set up with huge expenditure from the government exchequer remaining unutilized is criminal and needs to be stopped forthwith.

API MANUFACTURING IN INDIA

As is clear from the previous sections, China is currently the world's largest manufacturer of API. Other countries, very few in numbers, manufacture API in smaller quantities. As detailed earlier, none of the other countries now entering the formulation industry will be able to enter into API manufacturing and even if they do, it will be impossible for them to reach a scale that will be economically viable or ensure the quality of API. Except China, the Indian industry is decades ahead of other emerging players and it will be difficult for the new players to catch up in the short run. Given the concerns about the quality of Chinese API and the growing disenchantment across the globe with Chinese policies, there is a golden opportunity and also a challenge for India to enter the API industry in a big way.

The demand for quality API and formulations, both in the domestic and international arena, is bound to grow in the near future. The opportunity to manufacture API in India will need to address two major challenges. Firstly, the scale of API manufacturing has to be large enough to ensure reduction in the cost and secondly, the API manufactured in India has to be superior in quality to displace sources of API of doubtful quality. The cost effectiveness and the superiority of the quality of Indian API have to be apparent and there should be no doubts about them.

Bringing down the manufacturing cost of bulk drugs and increasing the global competitiveness of the domestic bulk drug industry, especially in the bulk drug manufacturing parks, by providing a number of common facilities, such as easy access to standard testing and infrastructure, had been visualized over a decade back. The details about the Hathi Committee and the Katoch Committee recommendations referred to above are pertinent in this context. The decision-making processes in the Government of India are excessively dilatory, and the pharmaceutical sector is replete with examples of tardiness in the decision-making processes. It also reflects that a sincere effort has not been made to comprehend the enormity of the opportunity that is waiting to be grabbed.

In the above perspective, no doubt, after recognizing the pharmaceuticals as a focus area in 2014, the Production Linked Incentive Schemes (PLI) for bulk drug parks, manufacturing of API and pharmaceuticals have been launched. However, there could be announced only in 2020. Judged by any standards, the period of six years spent for designing the schemes is far too long and what is worse is that these have been met with lukewarm response owing to their faulty design.

The PLI scheme announced in 2020 for bulk drug parks proposes to provide access to world-class common infrastructure facilities and common waste management system for API manufacturing units located in such parks. The scheme seeks to make India self-reliant for manufacturing API by increasing the competitiveness of the domestic industry. The scheme, as per the assessment of the government, is expected to lead to some optimization of resources and economies of scale.

As part of the scheme, three bulk drugs parks – with a total outlay of Rs. 3000 crore – are proposed to be developed in the country. The cap for an individual park has been kept at Rs. 1000 crore. The scheme has been operationalized from 2020–21 and will continue till 2024–25. It provides a one-time grant for common infrastructure facilities, which will be restricted to 70% of the project cost. The North Eastern States and the Hilly states will be provided assistance up to 90%. The assistance will be made available in four installments. Complete details in this regard are available on the website of the Department of Pharmaceuticals.[7]

With a view to reduce the import dependence in case of critical APIs, the central government has also launched the PLI Scheme for promotion of domestic manufacturing of critical KSM/DI/API in India. The financial outlay of the scheme has been pegged at Rs. 6940 crore, and it will remain operational from 2020–21 to 2029–30. The details of the scheme have been notified in the official Gazette of the government dated July 21, 2020. The scheme intends to boost domestic manufacturing of identified KSM, DI and API by attracting large investments in the sector with a view to reduce India's import dependence for critical APIs.

Under the scheme, financial incentives are proposed to be given based on sales made by selected manufacturers for 41 products for six years. For fermentation-based products, incentive would be 20% for the Financial Years 2023–24 to 2026–27, 15% for 2027–28 and 5% for 2028–29. For chemical synthesis-based products, incentive would be 10% for FY 2022–23 to FY 2027–28. Support under the scheme will be provided only to manufacturers of identified critical KSM/DI and API that have been registered in India. The details in this regard are also available on the website of the Department of Pharmaceuticals.[8]

The four segments into which the eligible KSM/API/DI have been divided include (i) key fermentation-based KSMs/DIs; (ii) niche fermentation-based KSMs/DIs; (iii) key chemical-based KSMs/DIs and (iv)other chemical synthesis-based KSM/DI/API. The scheme stipulates that the net worth of the applicant should not be less than 30% of the total committed investment. The proposed value addition has been pegged at

---

7. https://pharmaceuticals.gov.in/sites/default/files/Scheme%20for%20Promotion%20of%20 Bulk%20Drug%20Parks_0.pdf; and
https://pharmaceuticals.gov.in/sites/default/files/Guidelines%20of%20the%20Scheme%20 Promotion%20of%20Bulk%20Drug%20Parks_1.pdf
8. https://pharmaceuticals.gov.in/sites/default/files/Gazettee%20notification%20 of%20bulk%20 drug%20schemes_0.pdf

90% and 70% for fermentation and chemical synthesis-based applicants respectively.

The PLI Scheme for the pharmaceuticals that will be implemented during the Financial Years 2020–21 to 2028–29 has also been launched by the central government.[9] Global Manufacturing Revenue (GMR) has been taken as the basis for enhancing the reach of the scheme. For availing the scheme, the prospective applicants have been classified in three groups *viz.* Group A with a GMR of pharmaceutical goods of more than or equal to Rs. 5,000 crore; Group B with a GMR between Rs. 500 crore to Rs. 5,000 crore; and Group C with a GMR of less than Rs. 500 crore. The last group will also include a sub-group for MSME industry to address their specific challenges and circumstances. The allocation of incentive among the target groups has been capped at Rs. 11,000 crore for Group A; Rs. 2,250 crore for Group B; and Rs. 1,750 crore for Group C.

The scheme will cover pharmaceutical goods under three categories *viz.* Category 1 will include biopharmaceuticals, complex generic drugs, patented drugs or drugs nearing patent expiry, cell-based or gene therapy drugs, orphan drugs, special empty capsules like hydroxypropyl methycellulose (HPMC),[10] Pullulan, enteric, etc., complex excipients and phyto-pharmaceuticals. Category 2 includes API/KSM/DIs; and Category 3 includes other drugs not covered under Category 1 and Category 2. These will mainly be repurposed drugs; auto immune drugs, anti-cancer drugs, anti-diabetic drugs, anti-infective drugs, cardiovascular drugs, psychotropic drugs, anti-retroviral drugs; and in-vitro diagnostic devices. The rate of incentive has been kept at 10% of incremental sales value for Category 1 and Category 2 products for the first four years, 8% for the fifth year and 6% for the sixth year of production under the scheme. For Category 3 products, it will be 5% for first four years, 4% for the fifth year and 3% for the sixth year of production.

---

9. Posted On 24 February 2021 3:46PM by PIB Delhi.
10. Used as an inactive ingredient in the pharmaceutical industry, Hydroxypropyl methycellulose (HPMC) is a coating agent and film-former.

The government needs to be complimented that it has at last clearly identified that bulk drugs manufacturing holds the key for ensuring the drug security of the country and the position of the Indian pharmaceutical sector as the supplier of reliable quality drugs to the world. It has now been recognized that the drug security of the country is dependent on the ability of the country to ensure un-interrupted supply of quality bulk drugs and also our capacity to upscale our manufacturing to meet emergency situations.

At the same time, there are a few critical concerns that should also have been addressed. Owing to these concerns, the first PLI scheme proved to be a failure. On analysis it has been noted that the incentives offered were too less to attract any large investment, that too in a Greenfield project. As a result, the response to this was quite lukewarm. The second PLI which saw better consultation with the stakeholders is an improvement over the first one. However, it still has concerns as summarized below.

The first is with regard to the availability of funds for the proposed schemes as the fund allocations are made as part of the annual budgets. One only hopes that the COVID-19 pandemic-induced shrinking of receipts of the central government would not affect the allocations adversely. The second is the continuity of the schemes over a longer period of time with such modifications as may be necessary to attract investors and quality manufacturers. Uncertain business environment is the last thing that would interest any investor. The third concern is with regard to the scale of the schemes. These are still not ambitious enough for a country of India's size and potential. The very meager amount of incentives offered may not trigger any major investment, especially in the Greenfield projects, and make Indian companies globally competitive. It would have been desirable to have focused discussions with the potential investors before finalizing the schemes with clarity about the deliverables.

The fourth concern is that no provisions has been made to address the issues related to chemical industry that will provide the raw material, solvents and KSM for the pharmaceutical sector. Unless this issue is addressed, the Indian pharmaceutical industry cannot become globally competitive. Fifthly, the key issue of DPCO being applied even in case of API has not been factored in. Sixthly, the selection of products for the PLI scheme could have been done better and perhaps with better coordination with the stakeholders concerned. The seventh concern is more in the nature of apprehension that the schemes do not get jeopardized by red tape and dilatory tactics of structures. The eighth concern is that the scheme does not make any provisions for encouraging and setting up of pharmaceutical machine manufacturing facilities in India to lower fixed costs, enable savings in forex and reduce the time to set up additional facilities.

The ninth concern relates to no provision having been made to bolster the logistics infrastructure for connecting the key pharmaceuticals hubs in the country in order to facilitate quick and cost-efficient movement of goods, including cold chain facilities. The tenth concern is that the scheme does not seek to address the challenge of proper storage and transportation of medical products despite the fact that the existing infrastructure for it is in shambles. Lastly, no effort has been made to surmount the issues of excessive environmental and other restrictions that force the Indian industry not to take up clinical research and clinical trials within the county and conduct them abroad.

PHARMACEUTICAL EDUCATION

India has excessively been enamored by its prowess of technical and scientific manpower, and the demographic dividend with the least focus on quality. It needs to be noted that the edge in the technical and scientific resources, if there is any, is too thin to be complacent, and the demographic dividend can be useful only if the quality of human resources is scaled up substantially and the country is in a position to engage the vast population in productive activities. Besides, the potential on its own does not yield a dividend and it needs to be converted into reality through a well-calibrated policy intervention. There are also serious issues with the quality of human resources that the Indian universities are churning out.

India has demonstrated its potential to be the low-cost global player in the knowledge-based products and the credit for this should, *inter alia*, be given to public policies pursued during the initial phase of independent India. These helped create some of the great institutions that the country has. These include the IITs, IIMs and ISRO, to name a few. The success stories of the IITs, IIMs, etc., could, however, not be replicated while creating and nurturing institutions such as National Institutes of Pharmaceutical Education and Research (NIPERs). These institutions, as is evident from the facts on the ground, have not been able to acquire the stature befitting their status as institutions of national importance. NIPERs had been set up to overcome the crunch of talent under the NIPER Act, 1998 – as amended in 2007 – and are mandated to nurture and promote quality and excellence in pharmaceutical education and research.

Pharmacy education plays a crucial role in the growth of the pharmaceutical sector in the country. India has the largest number of trained pharmacy professionals in the world. The number of students graduating from pharmaceutical institutions in India is almost 14 times the number of students graduating in the USA in pharmaceutical sciences. In addition to this, medical practitioners and specialists also bring in a significant degree of expertise to clinical research and clinical trials. However, the quality of education imparted in many pharmacy colleges and universities in India is not up to the mark.

Since there is a major gap between the college curriculum and industry's requirements, most of the students passing out of these colleges and universities are not ready to take up even the existing roles in the industry, not to speak of donning the emerging roles that would become available with growing sophistication. The institutions still continue with the 20th century curriculum. Advanced skills in India are scarce as the number of students going in for research is limited. In fact, the percentage of those engaged at doctoral and postdoctoral levels is much lower in India as compared with the USA.

NIPER, Mohali was the first to be established and to begin with, it had done reasonably well in the initial years. The central government accorded in principle approval to set up six new NIPERs at Hyderabad, Ahmedabad, Kolkata, Guwahati, Raebareli and Hajipur in August 2007. These started functioning from the academic session 2007–08. The NIPERs were expected to innovate and train teachers in the field of pharmaceutical sciences, support creation of new knowledge and also develop a multi-disciplinary approach to undertake research and train manpower for high-end jobs in the pharmaceutical sector.

In the context of the role expected to be performed by them, it would be educative to read Report No. 3 of 2020 of the Comptroller and Auditor General of India.[11] The report brings out that none of the six new NIPERs had their own campus, and the posts of teaching and non-teaching staff had not been sanctioned by the Department of expenditure. In most cases, the land for their campuses had not been acquired and, in others, either the construction had not started or had been delayed. The NIPERs continue to function from the premises of mentor institutions and largely contractual staff has been engaged for teaching. Even in case of NIPER, Mohali, a large number of posts are lying vacant and the entire recruitment process has been embroiled in controversy. Invariably, there has been a huge delay in filling up of the posts, including those of Directors of NIPERs. Even the Board of Directors of six new NIPERs had not been constituted for many years.

NIPERs, which are institutions of national importance just in the same manner as IITs and IIMs are, were expected to have all necessary resources at their disposal. The facts brought out in the audit report do not paint a rosy picture. What is surprising is that three more NIPERs are now proposed to be established. If this is the position of the institutions of national importance, the state of affairs in other institutions can very well be imagined. There is clearly a dearth of resources at the disposal of NIPERs, the implementation is lax and the government commitment is conspicuous by its absence. The NIPERs are nowhere close to be the leading global

---

[11.] Available at: https://cag.gov.in/uploads/download_audit_report/2020/7)%20Chapter%202-of-3-2020-union-05f808dc1325eb4.40534448.pdf

institutions for learning and research in the field of pharmaceuticals. They are still not able to contribute in any significant manner to the furtherance of the objectives for which these had been set up in the first instance. These institutions follow the typical trajectory of many other Indian institutions that had been set up with a lot of fanfare but have been starved of necessary resources.

Life Sciences Sector Skill Development Council (LSSSDC) has been working on bridging the gap in skill-sets; however, its focus so far has been on preparing the manpower for routine and existing roles in the industry, rather than for taking up high-end jobs. Education in pharmaceutical sciences and related fields needs to be improved substantially for providing fully equipped human resources to the industry on a sustainable basis.

MOVING BEYOND GENERICS

India's dream of becoming the real pharmacy of the world can be realized only if the concerns, most of which have already been identified, are addressed to the satisfaction of all stakeholders and the industry fast-tracks beyond manufacturing generics and commences manufacturing specialized high-value and high-quality products and quality API. This would entail taking steps for attracting global investment, streamlining education and research, finding ways to fund R&D and taking up long-term risky projects, improving industry–academia collaboration, establishing a strong innovation ecosystem and finally, international collaborations, especially with the leading global players. All these require proactive action on the part of the industry and the government. Addressing environmental impediments and a PLI scheme for drug discovery and development also appear to be the need of the hour.

In brief, the pharmacy of the world is, at present, still quite a distance away from realizing its true potential. It will be necessary to overcome all the identified hurdles. It needs to be recognized that the competition is fast catching up. The only hope for the Indian pharmaceutical industry will be the quality of the product and that too at competitive prices. India is better placed to ward off the competition. However, if the quality of API/KSM and the human resources is not improved urgently, it will be impossible to manufacture the best-quality API and formulations, and innovate and develop new products. In order to incentivize the industry to enhance investment and production in diversified product categories, well-designed and suitably targeted interventions will be necessary to incentivize specific high-value goods such as biopharmaceuticals, complex generic drugs, patented drugs or drugs nearing patent expiry and cell based or gene therapy products, etc.

In the past, the decision-making processes have been slow and the schemes such as PLI have taken decades to be formulated. PLI schemes announced by the government in 2020 are a step in the right direction, but *prima facie* this appears to be a case of still being too conservative and too little and may be a little too late also. A grand plan, formulated after intense consultations with the prospective investors/industry that could take care of more concerns would have been desirable. The government will also need to have a consistent policy framework over a longer period of time and learn from the aggressive economic policies and directions provided by governments to the industry in countries such as Taiwan and South Korea, forcing both economies to perform beyond their capacity. The huge gap between the loud proclamations of intent, availability of resources and the actual delivery on the ground will also need to be bridged.

CHAPTER 10

INDIA – A MANUFACTURING HUB FOR MEDICAL DEVICES?

MEDICAL DEVICESAND HEALTHCARE

Before embarking upon the subject of this chapter, a little clarification will be in order. The present work includes medical devices as these devices and medicines together constitute a critical component of healthcare services. The development and availability of high-speed and high-precision diagnostic and improved therapeutic medical devices has brought about a paradigm shift in healthcare provisioning. The innovations have impacted human lives more than any other single factor and made it possible to render efficient healthcare services to patients with a range of products and services that would have been unthinkable even a decade back. The use of artificial intelligence, big data and different non-invasive techniques has improved the complexity and accuracy of screening and treating diseases, and many life-saving procedures have now become commonplace. Technological innovations have also made it possible to remotely monitor patients. The errors in diagnosis and treatment have been minimized resulting in better prevention, rehabilitation and recuperation.

To underline the criticality of medical devices, one can do no better than to recapitulate the WHO's assessment of medical devices. It states that in the absence of medical devices, it would be nearly impossible to carry out many simple medical procedures in managing healthcare, ranging from bandaging a sprained ankle to diagnosing HIV/AIDS or implanting an artificial hip. Improving access to appropriate medical devices is, as such, a crucial component of healthcare. Availability, accessibility, appropriateness and affordability have been identified as crucial '4 As' of medical devices by the WHO.[1] Non-invasive technologies or minimally invasive treatment options that became available as a result of the extensive use of medtech have revolutionized health care. It has now made treatment options available for those who would otherwise have been left untreated. One such example is Mitra Clip trans-catheter mitral valve repair therapy used in primary or secondary mitral regurgitation. Other examples include devices such as Impella pump used to pull the blood from the ventricle and push it out into the aorta for delivering oxygen-rich blood to the body while the heart rests and the doctor performs the Percutaneous Coronary Intervention or angioplasty with stent.

In the light of the facts brought out above, leaving medical devices out of the present work would not have been justified. Further, in India, medical devices continue to be included in the definition of drugs. On the other hand, medical devices being an important aspect of healthcare management deserve a much more detailed analysis and possibly, a separate book. The effort in the present chapter is, therefore, to capture only the most pertinent facets of medical devices, especially those relating to promotion of manufacturing and regulatory controls. For this reason, many aspects, including research, development and innovation, find only a perfunctory reference in this work.

SCOPE OF MEDICAL DEVICES

Medical devices industry is a multiproduct industry, comprising a wide range of engineering products used in the delivery of healthcare. Close to 15,000 medical devices are currently in use globally. New and innovative products could include adding new or additional features in the existing products or developing a new product altogether through disruptive technologies for addressing the felt needs of users and improving their experience. Keeping in view its usage, each medical device is unique.

[1.] Medical devices: managing the Mismatch, An outcome of the Priority Medical Devices project (https://apps.who.int/iris/bitstream/handle/10665/44407/9789241564045_eng.pdf)

Medical devices can be divided in to some broad categories such as: (i) Disposables & Consumables, including needles and syringes, etc; (ii) Surgical Instruments & Implants; (iii) Equipment & Electronics, including diagnostic imaging (MRI, X-Ray, Ultrasounds, etc); (iv) Dental Products such as dentures, braces, etc.; (v) Orthopedics and Prosthetics such as knee implants, artificial joints; (vi) Patient Aids, including hearing aids and pacemakers, etc. and (vii) Diagnostic Reagents.

GROWING MARKET FOR MEDICAL DEVICES

The range of medical devices being used in healthcare delivery and their sophistication is increasing with each passing day. A vast population in India that is still growing, coupled with a steady rise in the per capita Gross Domestic Product, has led to a sharp increase in the demand for medical devices and diagnostics in India. India is one of the top 20 global medical device markets of the world and the fourth largest in Asia. The domestic demand for medical devices is bound to grow multi-fold in the future as the country inches towards better healthcare and the standard of living of the public in general improves, with growing prosperity but along with increasing disease burden.

During the past two decades, the global surge in the demand for medical devices has been steeper than the increase in the demand for them in India. Improved availability, accessibility and affordability of medical devices of appropriate quality will further boost the demand and bring about a qualitative improvement in the delivery of healthcare services. The higher cost of medical devices, coupled with fast obsolescence, dampens the demand and restricts access to them. This is more so in less-developed countries where lower disposable incomes force the individuals to forego the use of medical devices rather than foregoing other necessities of life. This underpins the need for mass production of medical devices and bringing down their cost in the same way generic medicines brought down the cost of drugs, and increased their access and affordability.

The availability of quality medical devices at an affordable price could, in the Indian context, be a crucial factor for improved health outcomes. The increasing incidence of non-communicable diseases and the increase in geriatric population will further fuel the demand for quality healthcare and medical devices, both at homes and in healthcare facilities.

OPPORTUNITY KNOCKS AT INDIA'S DOORS

The intersection of technological innovations, entrepreneurship and demographic dividend presents an unprecedented opportunity and opens a new window for substantial augmentation of medical device manufacturing in India. 'Made in India' medical devices could be the global flavor in view of the hiatus involving China in the aftermath of the COVID-19-induced trade wars between the USA and China, along with the willingness of many large manufacturers to move out of China. Though this window is available for the manufacturing industry in general, the medical products are certainly the most lucrative ones. As India is also a preferred destination for medical tourism, at least for some countries, with the up gradation of the quality of medical products, the market for medical products and medical tourism could expand exponentially.

For a variety of reasons, the domestic medical devices industry in India is still confined largely to production of low-cost devices, a few implants and a much lesser number of radiology and ultrasound products, cathlabs and linear accelerators. Nearly 65% of around 800 domestic medical device manufacturers in India cater to consumables that are used largely for meeting domestic requirements with limited exports. Large multinationals, on the other hand, are engaged in providing medical devices requiring high-end technology.

Despite the often-touted scientific and engineering prowess of the country and the demographic dividend, close to 75% of medical devices required in India still continue to be imported. Most of such imports are from the USA, Germany, China, Singapore and the Netherlands. Electronics equipment forms the largest component of the Indian imports. Other imported medical devices include surgical instruments, implants, IVD reagents, disposables and consumables. *The very high level of dependence on the imported medical devices entails an annual outgo of around Rs. 45,000/-crore. This is bound to increase further with the passage of time.* As discussed elsewhere India has huge unemployment and underemployment and the demographic dividend is getting wasted. This offers a unique opportunity for the Indian medtech industry to seize the moment.

Quality medical devices that are affordable are needed to improve healthcare globally. Catering to the global market through economies of scale can help India in becoming the global manufacturing hub for medical devices. Incrementalism or inward-looking attitude would only thwart the mission. Achieving it will help generate employment, increase GDP and enhance the accessibility of medical devices across the globe. This will, however, need recalibrating India's response.

No time will be better than now for a decisive action to upscale the domestic medical devices industry and catapult it to an unassailable position globally. Opportunity knocks but once and as providence would have it, India is getting a second one. The Indian industry and the government have to take the chance willingly that could, with proper planning and execution, turn out to be the game changer.

ANALYSIS OF INDIA'S PREPAREDNESS

Can India rise to the occasion; can it be the medical devices manufacturing hub for the world or will it be a mere pipe dream? There cannot be any straightforward answer to these questions. However, an attempt can be made by breaking down the problems to components and carrying out an analysis. The pertinent questions in the process could be whether:

(i) India has the potential to become the global manufacturing hub for medical devices?

(ii) the country has the appetite or the will to scale up its medical devices industry to the global level?

(iii) the country has the required ecosystem in terms of infrastructure, supportive financial/fiscal and technical architecture and regulatory structures for taking up the challenge?

(iv) the appetite backed by sufficient follow-up action or to put it differently, is India capable of taking the requisite steps to scale up its ecosystem and provide sufficient incentives to attract medical devices industry?

INDIA'S POTENTIAL TO SCALE UP

There could be no doubt that India has the obvious advantage, especially in terms of the lower comparative cost of manufacturing in view of the demographic dividend, lower wages and availability of technical manpower. There is also no dearth of entrepreneurship amongst Indians. Many Indians have built and are running their businesses around the world successfully and many Indians are even steering some of the largest businesses globally. India has a distinct advantage in information technology and could possibly, with some extra effort, do so in the domain of artificial intelligence and machine learning as well. In theory, it would not be incorrect to surmise that India has the requisite potential and it could propel its medical device industry on to a high-growth trajectory with a compound annual growth rate (CAGR) of around 23% for the next ten years.

The CAGR projection is based on the fact that even without any substantial improvement in the ecosystem, the Indian medical device market nearly doubled from US$ 2.02 billion to US$ 3.9 billion at a CAGR of 15.8% between 2009 and 2015.[2] This prognosis is, however, subject to a number of things, including a whole lot of changes in the way we do business and also suitable augmentation of the skill sets of human resources. The large-scale expansion of the Indian medical device industry can be feasible only by catering to the global requirements and by increasing

---

[2.] Suchita Markhan *et al.* Indian Medical Device Sector- Blue Print & Regulatory Policy Roadmap, International Journal of Drug Regulatory Affairs.2020; 8(2): Also available online at https:// -IIDRA.com

and democratizing access to medical devices globally. For this, enhancing affordability through substantially reduced prices without compromising the quality will be necessary.

INDIA'S WILL TO SCALE UP

This brings us to the second question. The knowledge about the opportunity to step up manufacturing of medical devices has been with the government and the industry for over a decade now. The matter has continued to engage the attention of the authorities concerned. Post COVID-19 developments have made it obvious. Briefly, it was in recognition of this that the medical devices manufacturing was identified as one of the 25 focus sectors under the 'Make in India' campaign in 2014. The Union Government had, in 2014, proclaimed itself as the government with a difference and had, in various pronouncements, indicated its intent to usher in transformational reforms through programs such as 'Make in India'. The avowed objective was to make India a global manufacturing hub by attracting the state-of-the-art technology and capital into the country.

Propelling the production of medical devices was also one of the core issues discussed by the group of secretaries year after year that continued to be set up by Prime Minister Modi. Presentations on the recommendations of these groups were made before the Prime Minister and his Cabinet colleagues every year. The medical devices sector had also reportedly figured prominently in the discussions at the highest level, including during the visit of the Prime Minister to the USA, *albeit* for reasons of allegedly arbitrary pricing practices in India and also against the medical devices being included in the definition of a drug that put the American manufacturers at a disadvantageous position.

Besides the efforts of the Union government, many state governments have, in the recent past, also demonstrated their strong desire for creating an ecosystem conducive for doing business and evinced interest in medical device manufacturing. These include Andhra Pradesh, Telengana, Tamil Nadu and Uttar Pradesh. There is a growing realization that the Indian medical device industry cannot realize its full potential by catering merely to the domestic demand; it has to scale up both quantitatively and qualitatively and meet the global demand in just the same manner that Indian generic drugs industry does in case of medicines.

DOES INDIA HAVE THE REQUIRED ECOSYSTEM?

Like any other industry, the Medtech industry needs good physical and other infrastructure, including railways, roads, airports and information technology; required human resources; the market for the product; financial/fiscal support that is comparable to the best in the world or even better; consistency and predictability about the governmental policies; and more important than anything else, the existence of a robust regulatory structure for certifying the quality of medical products. Absence of all or anyone of these elements would have a negative bearing on the attractiveness of a country as a manufacturing hub for medical devices.

Currently in many parts of the country, the infrastructure is still not up to the mark and there are also serious concerns with regard to both the connectivity and the law and order. Efforts are, however, being made by many states to improve the ground situation and in the recent past, there has been a healthy competition between the states. Luckily, India does not have the dearth of human resources and the required skilling is something doable, even in the short run. It will, however, be important to note that human resources which are otherwise a great asset, could turn into a massive liability the moment these resources are not constructively engaged in productive activities.

A large segment of India's population is currently unemployed and as such, the country is not able to benefit from favorable demography. Further, the dividend needs to be utilized while it is available and with the efflux of time, it will wane. As far as the market is concerned, as stated earlier, India has a large market and it is increasing rapidly. The Indian medical devices industry could cater to the global market subject to concerns regarding quality being addressed satisfactorily.

Despite recognition of the fiscal/financial incentives needed for hastening the growth of the medical devices industry in India, little has been done to work out a suitable package to address the concerns of the medical devices industry. If anything, the concerns in this regard have only grown. In this connection, the details mentioned in the later paragraphs that highlight the gist of a combined presentation made in July 2016 in the PMO by all the medical devices manufacturing associations, action taken thereon and the new production linked incentive scheme to support manufacturing of medical devices and provide production linked incentive to the industry are relevant.

It needs to be clearly understood that if India has to be the global player in the field of medical devices, the country needs to first set its house in order, and this order will comprise many intertwined factors, including encouraging the domestic industry to scale up and be prepared for conforming to regulatory and voluntary standards demanded by the discerning global consumer.

There will also be a need to provide attractive packages for the global industry to relocate to India. It is not uncommon to note that the procurement policies followed by the governments, both the central and the state, put a lot of impediments in the way of domestic manufacturers as they are not assured of the quality in view of lax compliance with regulatory and voluntary standards by the Indian industry. For example, while the imported medical devices with CE mark are welcome, in case of domestic manufacturers, unreasonable requirements such as proving conformance through clinical trials, etc., are stipulated. For the same reason, the procurement process also gives preference to USFDA-approved devices.

Consistency and predictability of the business environment, especially the elements having a bearing on the profitability of the industry over a longer period of time, holds the key for attracting investment. This has been one of the weakest areas of the Indian governance architecture whether on account of change in the ruling political party or due to pressures of vote bank politics. Without going into too many details, the decisions such as retrospective taxation by the Centre or change in the policies by the

Andhra Government after the new government headed by YS Jaganmohan Reddy of Yuvajana Sramika Rythu Congress Party (YSRCP) came to power, demonstrate this aspect very clearly. Undoubtedly, there has to be a long-term policy that does not undergo sudden change for any reason, and the industry should be able to predict what the policy entails in the longer run while deciding to invest in the country.

As far as the Indian regulatory structures are concerned, the less said the better. While details in this regard have already been recapitulated in earlier chapters, it is enough to say that in the absence of a stringent regulatory structure, there has been a move to go in for voluntary certification so that the medical devices can be exported. More details in this regard have been given in the succeeding sections. As in the case of drugs, the division of responsibility across the departments of the Government of India and the dual control of the central and state governments, provides a sure recipe for disaster.

NURTURING ECOSYSTEM

The Indian experience in implementation of the plans and strategies has not been very encouraging and, more often than not, India has botched it up. To put it plainly, in India there is a huge gap between defining (identifying) the problem (issue); identifying an optimal solution to solve the identified problem; and implementing of the identified solution at the ground level. Even when the problem has been defined correctly, the solutions proffered are invariably sub-optimal and the implementation is poor. The situation is further worsened by tardy implementation by the machinery at the ground level. This has been the story of many plans that were in theory, as many would argue, exceptional and outstanding, but were marred by poor implementation. Though the counterview is that any plan or policy that is divorced from ground reality and does not factor in impediments, can yield only sub-optimal results.

While noting the limitations of governmental structures to deliver, credit must, however, be given where it is due. Some positive steps had been initiated during the first five years of the NDA government from May 2014 to 2019. These include permitting up to 100% foreign direct investment under the automatic route for manufacturing medical devices, partial rationalization of customs duty structure to remove the inverted duty structure and framing of the Medical Devices Rules, 2017 that spell out the regulatory framework for medical devices for the first time. Though these rules do not make good the absence of the parliamentary law on the subject, these are in conformity with the Global Harmonization Task Force framework and best international practices.

The Bureau of Indian Standards has done a commendable work in laying down the standards for medical devices. The setting up of the Andhra Medtech Zone in Vishakhapatnam demonstrates that scaling up is feasible. The separate legislation for regulating medical devices did not materialize despite the fact that a draft Medical Devices (Regulation) Bill had been finalized long time back.. NITI Aayog has also gone into the issue, but the legislation is nowhere on the horizon. Even other regulatory reforms have largely come to a grinding halt.

Though significant, the steps taken so far are not sufficient for a complete transformation of the Indian Medtech industry. In the absence of a legislative framework and concrete measures to attract industry, these look like a false start. Similarly, the promise of a separate vertical within the CDSCO to deal with medical devices regulation did not materialize.

Sufficient follow-up action has not been taken in pursuance of the 2014 announcement designating medical devices sector as a focus area. Consequently, there is a huge gap between the intent and the action taken. An objective assessment of the performance of the government will indicate that India has not been able to think big and has always been engrossed in trivialities and procedures owing largely to the lack of appreciation of the ground reality. It has starved the organizations/institutions rather than converting them into revenue-yielding instrumentalities of the state. Red tape has, owing to its fears, ruled the roost in the absence of the political executive's capacity to take care of policy formulation.

Needless to say, the fossilized structures that are, amongst others, scared of the three Cs *viz.* the Central Bureau of Investigation, the Central Vigilance Commission and the Comptroller & Auditor General of India, have failed to deliver.

Global reach presupposes global quality. Currently nothing concrete has been done to address the serious concerns about the quality of products, data integrity, etc., for which the Indian generic drugs industry has been facing the flak for quite some time.

INDUSTRY PRESENTATION IN THE PMO

During June–July 2016, a series of meetings of all associations of medical device manufacturers were arranged in the MoHFW to evolve an agreed action plan to take the 'Make in India' initiative forward in case of medical devices. All major associations of medical device manufacturers, staff of the CDSCO and the staff in the Ministry worked painstakingly everyday till late in the night and also on all holidays, Saturdays and Sundays for finalizing an agreed action plan for positioning India amongst the top five medical device manufacturing countries in the world.

Given the divergence of opinion amongst different industry associations on key issues, bringing them on the same platform and coming out with a comprehensive and viable plan of action was a major challenge. However, everyone was charged up and keen on burying the differences in the larger interests of the country and medical devices industry. Based on the agreed action plan, a detailed presentation was made before the Principal Secretary to the Prime Minister on July 11, 2016 in South Block, in which five industry associations and officials from the Ministries concerned were present.

The presentation highlighted that if India had to achieve universal healthcare, it has to be ensured that the five pillars of healthcare *viz.* the healthcare providers (hospitals); the pharmaceutical industry; the medical devices industry; the diagnostic industry and health insurance industry, grew in tandem. It was emphasized that although being the smallest amongst these five areas, the medical devices sector was a critical contributor for improving the healthcare outcomes in the country through affordable and innovative low-cost delivery models.

The presentation brought out that India possessed the pre-requisites for ushering in a fast-paced growth of the sector, provided the identified constraints could be overcome. These included availability of the basic medical technologies in most cases and, to some extent, advanced and the state-of-the-art medical technologies for addressing patient needs; medical infrastructure comparable to the best in the world in some cases; linguistic skills and the capacity to absorb advanced technology. Given these factors, medtech was, during the presentation, propositioned as an attractive option for India.

It was indicated that India had a large domestic market that was still growing and India enjoyed the comparative cost advantage. It was stated that sub-market fragmentation due to variations on account of area/specialty, geography and clinical processes might blunt the advantage to some extent, but this could be overcome without difficulties. The associations highlighted that starting relatively late, India needed to leapfrog many other countries with attractive and globally competitive, focused and consistent policy to provide sufficient impetus for growth of the sector in the long run.

The presentation underlined that there was a need to work on both demand and supply fronts. On the demand side, it was recommended that the domestic market will need to be enlarged, including through modernization of medical education, increasing expenditure on health and higher pace of technology adoption. On the supply side, a slew of measures encompassing the regulatory, infrastructural, financial and skill-set up gradation were proposed to counter manufacturing and R&D competition from China, Singapore, Malaysia, Ireland, Puerto Rico, etc.

It was pointed out that with respect to the supply side issues, both short- and long-term interventions will be needed and demand side management can be possible only in the long run. Industry associations advocated for evolving a comprehensive policy for medical devices and suggested establishment of a special purpose vehicle for inter-departmental cohesion and management of international relationships.

Specific recommendations encompassing financial, infrastructural, regulatory, skill development and demand generation were brought out during the presentation. The suggested financial measures included abolition of corporate tax for medical devices; provision of export concessions; 100% capex subsidy on technology transfer; tax holiday for 5–7 years; subsidized and expeditious registration and weighted tax deduction up to 200% on R&D investments. It also advocated accelerated depreciation of 200%; 5% interest subvention and re-imbursement of 50% of the certification fee charged by CE and the USFDA to startups in niche categories. Favorable tariff in case of raw materials, consumables and retention of the then prevalent import duty on finished medical devices were also advocated.

Other recommendations made during the presentation included cluster-based development of common facilities with governmental support; expansion of IVDs/medtech products from DBT/DST/BIRAC/CSIR, etc.; establishment of quality testing and validation labs and common photo and 3D printing facilities, machining centers, metallurgy units and molding facilities, along with adequate cold chain, modern warehousing, and packaging and sterilization logistics on the infrastructural front.

On the regulatory side, a separate law to regulate medical devices and the medical devices not being subjected to pharmaceutical style pricing; measures to ensure single use of medical devices and implementation of the measures already identified for enhancing ease of doing business, etc., were proposed. Promotion of joint ventures to ensure transfer of the state-of-the-art technology and incentivizing high-end tech transfer and adoption through targeted imports and rationalizing public procurement by treating the CDSCO approvals at par with the USFDA/CE approvals were highlighted as urgent requirements. It was also mentioned that the CDSCO needed to have a full-fledged medical device vertical or alternatively, a separate regulatory authority may be set up for regulation of medical devices.

The longer-term measures suggested included increasing the expenditure on public healthcare to 3% of the GDP, prioritization of medical devices on the basis of local disease prevalence and associated severity, and increasing awareness about adoption of technology; creation of world-class R&D and innovation facilities; expeditious commercialization of R&D outcomes and creation of an equity fund of Rs. 5000 crore for investment in priority areas such as pre-testing and animal labs, including bovine/porcine animal labs for pre-clinical studies; creation of centers of excellence in different institutions and encouraging cross-functional knowledge sharing.

Senior PMO officials were, however, not interested in discussing such major policy prescriptions and shifted the entire discussion to sorting out smaller bottlenecks in the regulatory arena, ostensibly in their zeal for showing impressive improvements in ease of doing business. Had a healthy deliberation on the issue commenced at that point of time, the country would have been better prepared to leverage the opportunity thrown up in the post COVID-19 scenario. The opportunity to evolve a coherent long-term vision and policy was sacrificed at the altar of short-term publicity. It was only in 2020 that some concrete steps have been initiated to address some of the issues identified a long time back.

MEDICAL DEVICES PARKS AND PRODUCTION LINKED INCENTIVE SCHEME

The government has now acknowledged that the medical devices sector in India suffers from a considerable cost of manufacturing disability *vis-à-vis* competing economies, *inter alia*, on account of lack of adequate infrastructure, domestic supply chain and logistics, high cost of finance, inadequate availability of power, limited design capabilities, low focus on R&D and skill development, etc.

With the objective of boosting domestic manufacturing, attracting large investment in the medtech sector, the central government had, in early 2020, launched a scheme for promotion of four medical devices parks across the country in which common infrastructure facilities are to be financed by the government up to an upper limit of Rs. 400 crore. A Production Linked Incentive (PLI) Scheme has also been approved for Promotion of Domestic Manufacturing of Medical Devices to ensure a level playing field for the domestic manufacturers with a total financial outlay of Rs.3420 crore for the period 2020–21 to 2027–28. These are some right steps in the desired direction. The guidelines of the PLI scheme were released in the month of July 2020.[3]

The scheme takes within its fold four target segments of medical devices *viz.* (i) Cancer care/Radiotherapy; (ii) Radiology & Imaging (both ionizing & non-ionizing radiation products); (iii) Anesthetics & Cardio Respiratory, including Catheters of Cardio Respiratory Category & Renal Care Needles; and (iv) All Implants, including implantable electronic devices. Linking the incentive to production measured through incremental increase in the year-on-year sales is also a major innovation of the scheme and definitely an improvement over the previous schemes, including M-SIPS of the Ministry of Electronics and Information Technology.

A detailed analysis of the scheme brings out that it may still not be sufficient to attract large-scale investments in the medical devices sector. The major limitations of the scheme include the very low incentive offered at 5% of incremental sales. The incentive has been kept uniform for all target segments and does not accord any preference to priority medical devices. Further, the incentive has been capped unrealistically low. If the target is to reach the global market, the scheme cannot be operated only to promote the small-scale industry. India needs large-scale investment in the sector as only economies of scale could enhance the global competitiveness of India's medical devices industry.

Consistency of policy is one of the most critical elements for attracting long- term investment. The scheme does not give an assurance of its continuation beyond the stipulated period. A doubt is also lingering in the minds of the many existing manufacturers whether the scheme would push them out of business with no increase in the overall manufacturing of medical devices and new manufacturers largely displacing the existing

---

[3.] Details available at: https://pharmaceuticals.gov.in/sites/default/files/Gazette%20 notification%20 of%20Medical% 20Device%20schemes_0.pdf

ones on account of higher incentives becoming available only to the new entrants.

Approval of the schemes may not mean much as funds for each scheme are provided through annual budgets, and while approved schemes will have a preferential claim, the actual availability of funds will, in most cases, vary from year to year. Thus, in case of the scheme for strengthening drug regulatory structures at a cost of Rs. 1750 crore in 2015, the annual budgetary allocations were much lower and less than one-third of the approved funds could be made available. One can only hope that the pandemic-induced financial constraints do not play havoc with this scheme.

The focus of the government so far has been on small and incremental changes, rather than structural and long-term strategic issues. Sporadic efforts to address the concerns are not only insufficient but also directionless. The scheme fails to visualize a big picture, with many uncertainties, including availability of required funds in the annual budgets. It must be conceded that some of the limitations of the scheme are known only now due to the benefit accruing from developments post the onset of COVID-19.

It would be appropriate to amend the scheme and peg the incentives at 15–25% of the incremental sales for the first ten years, with higher incentives for critical/priority areas and taper it down to 5–10% for ten years beyond that. The ceiling on the quantum of incentives to attract economies of scale needs to be removed and investors incentivized for induction of latest technology by offering attractive subsidy on new state-of-the-art machinery that takes the environmental concerns into account. The window to avail the incentives should be kept open for a longer period of time to ensure proper planning and execution by potential investors after assessing the pros and cons.

The current rates of GST on domestic medical devices may be brought down to zero for the next ten years and the customs duty on finished or semi-finished medical devices be doubled every four years. Quality concerns may be addressed by constituting a special task force to suggest necessary changes/augmentation of structures engaged in regulating quality of medical devices. Capital expenditure for establishment of common services facilities should be fully funded by the central government and the cost should not be capped at Rs. 400 crore. The benefit of lower cost should be passed on to the manufacturers by allowing only the variable cost to be recovered with reasonable profit. As discussed elsewhere, India has huge unemployment and underemployment and the demographic dividend is being wasted. This offers a unique opportunity for the Indian medtech industry to seize the moment.

RESEARCH AND DEVELOPMENT

R&D is a key element for attaining the leadership position in the field of medical technology. This will entail massive investments in terms of personnel, money and material including for augmenting the skill sets of the students in the technical institutions. Those graduating from at-least the institutions of national importance must have the capacity to don roles in the cutting edge technologies. India is definitely not in a position to spare a lot of resources for research, development and innovations and, therefore, aligning India's R&D with the developed world could be beneficial to both.

The Department of Biotechnology has launched an Industry–Academia Collaborative Mission for accelerating discovery research for early development of biopharmaceuticals in India for empowering biotech entrepreneurs and accelerating the development of high-quality and affordable products through cutting-edge technologies. Being managed under the aegis of Biotechnology Industry Research Assistance Council, a not-for-profit organization, R&D projects with respect to medical devices are also covered under this project. Though the quantum of funding given for this is very low, it is an initiative in the right direction.

Addressing restrictions imposed from the environmental angle need to be eased to ensure more pre-clinical research and clinical trials. It would also be desirable to list out the public facilities that can be utilized for undertaking research & development, testing, etc. by the private sector on payment of a nominal fee. For the IVD, the government must consider positioning an institute such as NIB to do hand-holding to ensure the industry gets world class assistance to scale up its activities in conformity with best global practices. Such hand-holding can make a material difference in the growth of IVD industry. This aspect has also been covered in detail in an earlier chapter.

REGULATION OF MEDICAL DEVICES

Medical devices that had been notified as drugs continue to be regulated by the national and state-level regulators on the pattern of medicines. A large number of medical devices, however, remain unregulated. In such cases, the certification by regulators of manufacturing countries continues to be accepted without any oversight by Indian regulators. This leaves a vital component of medical products virtually unregulated. Further, the CDSCO and state regulators are still manned by professionals drawn mainly from the pharmaceuticals field. It is not to say that they are not competent; nonetheless, their core competence is not in the field of medical devices or engineering products.

Keeping in view the severe limitations of manpower as well as expertise, a proposal had been floated on the basis of the Satyananda Mishra Committee to create separate verticals in the CDSCO, and one of the proposed verticals was to exclusively look after the regulation of medical devices. The details of how the proposal was scuttled have been included in an earlier chapter.[4] Another component of the proposal for creation of posts at lower levels was separately processed for approval of the Finance Minister. As explained earlier, that proposal helped in creation of only a few posts.

The idea to have a separate regulator for medical devices has been floated from time to time. This, however, appears to be absurd and not worth being pursued. Both good-quality drugs and medical devices are integral components of healthcare management, and there are a large number of products that do not strictly fit in the binary of either a medical

---

[4.] See Chapter 3 for details.

device or a drug. The WHO cites the example of a syringe prefilled with a medicinal product and a catheter coated with heparin to prevent blood clotting as two examples of such products.

The Indian medical devices manufacturers have continued to push for regulation of all devices. The absence of regulation impacts export of medical devices to many countries despite sufficient demand. Industry has been demanding that all medical devices be regulated and the system of notification of individual devices as drugs for being regulated be given up. The industry has been proposing that medical devices should be defined with clarity so that any product which falls within its definition is automatically brought under regulation and does not need to be notified individually.

With respect to imports, a lot of rebranding and relabeling takes place and, in the process, pre-owned equipment find their way into India. A large number of such equipment are obsolete and are imported into the country in the name of cheap imports, affordability and better access. During the COVID-19 pandemic, the unscrupulous elements have been seen gunning for the kill. The ventilators that are 15–20 years old and have been imported from dubious sources and refurbished multiple times by non-qualified local technicians have been sold for Rs. 4–6 lakh a piece. Such a compromise on the quality of medical devices also gets condoned in the absence of a robust regulatory structure. On the other hand, the current system of procurement of medical equipment, including ventilators, is non-transparent and in the absence of laid-down mandatory standards, even the governmental agencies insist on USFDA-approved or CE- marked medical devices. This dampens the domestic industry as it is compelled to seek certification from external certification bodies at a huge expenditure.

For years, the demand of the industry for more and efficient regulation of medical devices was not addressed. Hence, the Association of Indian Medical Device Industry (AIMED), in collaboration with the Quality Council of India and the National Accreditation Board for Certification Bodies, rolled out a voluntary quality certification scheme to fill the regulatory vacuum for quality certification of medical devices in the country (ICMED) on March 15, 2016, coinciding with the World Consumer Day. It aims at establishing product credentials and instilling confidence amongst buyers, as well as enhancing patient safety and providing better consumer protection. It remains a voluntary quality certification scheme for medical devices and is intended to reduce trading of substandard products or devices of doubtful origins. It seeks to bring down the time and cost of obtaining globally accepted quality certification for Indian companies and eliminate the malpractices of substandard or fraudulent certification or quality audits.

Another important aspect that should be addressed at this stage expeditiously is to establish a synergy between the CDSCO, QCI and BIS with a view to evolving standards for regulation of medical devices and harmonized action for ensuring quality of medical devices.

RESPONSIBILITY OF MANUFACTURERS AND SUPPLIERS

The healthcare sector has, during the last couple of decades, undergone a metamorphosis due to continuous technological advancement, leading to availability of a diverse range of medical devices. It is critical that medical devices conform to quality standards and requirements in view of the growing complexity and precision required in healthcare delivery. Any compromise in quality could have devastating consequences for public health. The responsibility of the manufacturers and suppliers has, in view of these developments, increased manifold for ensuring conformance with laid-down quality parameters for manufacturing, warehousing, documentation and traceability. Each manufacturer and market authorization holder should, therefore, establish robust in-house quality control and quality assurance structures.

In light of the facts brought out in this chapter, the action points could be summarized under the following categories:

(a) expeditiously review all the schemes and come out with a modified mega plan to make India the global medical devices manufacturing hub

(b) strengthen medical products regulatory and surveillance mechanism, including through enactment of suitable legislation and framing rules and provision of additional qualified manpower

(c) come out with a comprehensive plan of action for augmentation of innovations and R&D in India

(d) establish synergy between the CDSCO and other bodies involved in standard setting

(e) provide hands-on support to industry by making the public facilities available for research, development, testing and analysis, and imparting training to professionals

(f) strengthen post marketing surveillance of medical devices and establish robust institutional arrangements for capturing and analyzing data

(g) engage civil society organizations/patient-based organizations for reporting adverse events

(h) establish synergy between standard setting bodies and CDSCO.

CHAPTER 11

THE CONCLUDING REMARKS

Human existence is much more than a mere survival or animal existence. The highest attainable standard of physical and mental health is a basic human right and an entitlement of every individual. As a sub-set and an integral part of the right to life, accessibility to and affordability of good-quality medical products is indispensable for enjoyment of this right. Non-availability of essential medical products, on the other hand, would not only violate this basic human right but could also snatch away the life itself. Every state has an obligation to ensure that each individual residing within its boundaries has an equal opportunity to enjoy the right to health and healthy living.

In the Indian context, the denial of essential medical products of good quality violates Article 21 of the Constitution of India that guarantees the right to life and liberty. It also militates against the Directive Principles of State Policy enumerated in Part IV of the Constitution of India.

In view of the above, the medical products – whether manufactured and traded for meeting domestic or global demand – should fully meet the prescribed standards. Conformance with international standards and instruments for medical products goes a long way in assuring their quality. Of course, ethnic and other differences need to be duly factored in while laying down standards. Expanding access to quality medicines and healthcare products is also one of the important objectives of the United Nations Sustainable Development Goals.

Globally, medical products not meeting the acceptable standards of quality, safety and efficacy continue to be a major health concern as failure of treatment on account of poor-quality products results in increased morbidity and mortality; gives rise to adverse drug events and causes antimicrobial resistance. Medical products of poor quality also erode public trust in national health systems; negate the right to health and, in many cases, run off with the life itself. On the other hand, the poor and vulnerable sections of the society across countries cannot afford costly medical products and are, in the process, denied the right to health.

The generic medicines manufactured in India, due to their lower cost, fill up a major vacuum in the global healthcare supply chain and enhance access to healthcare. Many Indian manufacturers successfully meet the most stringent quality requirements specified by regulators of importing countries. There are, however, serious concerns about the quality of many other manufacturers. The product quality is not a given constant and it continues to evolve, with additional requirements being added with the passage of time and accretion of new knowledge. In order to continue to play a dominant role, the Indian pharmaceutical industry needs to respond effectively to additional requirements that crop up from time to time.

Till now, only a few medical devices are regulated in India, and the majority of them still remain unregulated. Medical devices are regulated as part of the drugs as these devices were not in use to any great extent when the law was enacted in 1940. Over the years, the usage of medical devices has gone up considerably, and currently it is difficult to visualize cure, treatment, recuperation or rehabilitation without medical devices.[1] With over 75% of the domestic requirement of medical devices being met through imports and domestic manufacturing being restricted largely to low-cost medical devices, the Indian medical devices industry is nowhere closer to its potential.

Concerns expressed by many regulators and countries about the quality of made in India medical products dent the claim of India to be the pharmacy of the world. The concerns are relatable to serious gaps in the constitutional and legal framework, and the inadequacies of institutional architecture that could not be addressed for decades despite recommendations of many

---

[1.] The comments of the WHO in Chapter 9 may be referred to in this context.

government-appointed committees.[2] The provisions of the Government of India Act, 1935 that gave disproportionate authority to the provinces; a few other fault-lines of the Indian Constitution, including with regard to the division of authority between the Centre and the states; prevalence of archaic laws, diffused regulatory structures and multiplicity of the departments and agencies that handle medical products with inadequate coordination between them; and serious flaws in implementation at the ground level contribute to the current state of affairs.

The efficiency of drug regulatory authorities in any country has a tremendous bearing on the quality of medical products. A modern, robust and efficient regulatory system for medical products, especially in countries supplying medicines globally, is a good investment in public health and also makes good business sense. The regulatory authority not only ensures the quality of medical products but also helps in fostering innovation. The authority, therefore, needs the best possible human resources, including experts in relevant specialties, and the state-of-the-art equipment for testing and analyzing medical products.

The current Indian regulatory arrangement for medical products defies all logic and is against the basic tenets of management as it makes multiple authorities with overlapping remits responsible for drug regulation. Multiple regulators (37 in total) and other authorities often work at cross purposes. It causes confusion and information asymmetry across layers of regulatory mechanism.

To a large extent, the state and central regulators in India operate independently, with minimal coordination amongst them through the ineffective mechanism of Drugs Consultative Committee, which meets far too infrequently and, in accordance with the current arrangements, could hardly be expected to make any meaningful contribution for better regulation of medical products. There are also serious concerns about the lack of expertise within the regulatory structures, especially in medtech,

---

[2.] Chapter 2 and 3 may be seen for details.

and new and emerging areas such as biologicals, stem cells and regenerative medicines.

The state regulatory authorities, the CDSCO, and other supporting institutions such as the NIB or IPC – all are crippled for want of resources. The CDSCO is critically dependent on multiple external mechanisms such as GEAC, RCGM, SECs, etc. The fact that the CDSCO does not have any in-house expertise, even for effectively coordinating the meetings of many expert committees, is problematic. The position of the state drug regulators is still worse as they are susceptible to pressures both from the political executive as well as the pharmaceutical industry and on account of inadequate manpower and expertise.

Many of the ills of the pharmaceutical sector in India are the consequence of this state of diffused responsibility. The resultant confusion and chaos create conditions conducive for corruption, rent seeking and other malpractices, both on the part of the regulators and the regulated. It also results in marketing of poor-quality drugs that are manufactured, stored, sold and administered to patients not only in India but globally as well. Some of the manufacturing happens in non-licensed and non-GMP-compliant facilities.

The ability to ensure effective enforcement of law is a major deterrent. Given the skeletal and diffused drug regulatory set-up in India, inspection of manufacturing units, wholesalers, distributors and others in the supply chain are few and far between. They are undertaken in an *ad hoc* manner and are mostly not premised on scientific lines. In most cases where inspections are carried out, no concrete action – administrative or otherwise – is taken for rectifying the lapses detected during inspections. In fact, the regulatory authorities do not have the required resources for any follow up action. The poor record-keeping and absence of data integrity has been the subject matter of criticism by the courts, the Parliament and the regulators of importing countries.

Unguided and arbitrary exercise of discretion by regulatory officials also leads to non-uniformity in law enforcement. While a large number of cases do not reach the prosecution stage, even in case of those that reach prosecution, the courts take their own sweet time to pronounce the verdict. Some database is now being built centrally about the various aspects concerning violation of related laws, and the sharing of information by state drug regulatory authorities. However, it remains voluntary. Many non-conforming activities continue to be ignored, which open the floodgates for more transgressions in manufacturing, storage, transportation and other processes related to medical products. Many foreign and multinational companies operating in India are also equally complicit and market products that are irrational, useless and harmful.

The policy of least cost being the main determinant for government procurements, irrespective of the quality of the product or their meeting basic requirements such as stability during the shelf-life of the product or bioequivalence with innovator products or even dissolution and other requirements being satisfied, has been a major reason for the proliferation of substandard and poor-quality products in the market. This explains the higher NSQ drugs in government supplies as compared with samples drawn from the market. Along with the pressure on price front by NPPA, the practice has also led to increased procurement of cheaper but poorer quality API from China. As a result, dependence on imported API/KSM/DI has gone up. Over 70% of API imports are from China, with other countries chipping in to a very small extent. This illustrates two things viz that healthcare is not a perfect market and excessive price controls could be counter-productive. In case of medicines, affordability cannot be at the cost of quality; it is not a case of 'either' 'or', and medical products must meet both. Quality medical products have to be affordable to the masses in general for enjoying the right to health.

The repeated transgressions by the manufacturers and the state drug regulators results in the influx of a large number of rational and irrational FDCs in the market. While initially no action was taken, the later efforts of the government were frustrated through judicial processes, and the irrational FDCs continue to be marketed even after the issues had been examined *de novo* by DTAB and its sub-committee as per the directions of the Supreme Court. Fresh cases have been filed in various High Courts who have granted stay in a number of cases.

The failure to come out with clear and timely policies, including the one with regard to the incentives for setting up of bulk drugs or medical devices parks in the country, has held back the API and medical technology industry from reaching its true potential. As a result, poor-quality raw materials and refurbished medical devices without proper evaluation and quality certification get dumped in India. The procurement-related issues with the insistence on USFDA-approved products result in non-utilization of the installed capacity in case of medical devices. Excessive price controls, including that of the API, are regressive.

Human resources management activities, including training of drug regulators, are largely unstructured and temporary. The processes of recruitment and appointment are time consuming and dilatory. Neglect of education in pharmaceutical and related areas has been a major stumbling block, and it has resulted in the scarcity of the required talent for employment in industry and research activities. NIPERs, the institutions of national importance, still continue to struggle with outsourced faculty and poor or no infrastructure. The sector skill development councils have only been able to evolve training programs for current routine functions and a lot of work for skilling for the cutting edge areas is still ignored.

The digital infrastructure such as *SUGAM* and *XLN* need further up gradation to facilitate hassle-free online transactions. The efficiency in case of recall of drugs should result in every single unit of the defective product being withdrawn from the supply chain, with a proper reconciliation of stocks manufactured, distributed and recalled. However, the recall processes in India are largely non-transparent. The efforts made so far either for reforming and strengthening the drug regulatory structures or promoting pharmaceutical and medical devices industry have failed as these were half-hearted, with inadequate makeover plans formulated without any careful assessment of the alternatives against a clear set of criteria for success; absence of ownership, especially at the level of political executive; non-alignment of the senior members of bureaucracy in directing, leading and monitoring the transformation; and last but not the least, inadequate engagement for on-boarding all stakeholders. The efforts made so far also did not succeed mainly because of bad design and the lack of sufficient attention to the rewiring of the legal and the organizational architecture. Implementation at ground level also remains a serious concern.

The rising sense of sub-nationalism fanned primarily by regional parties and the competition between states to attract industry, even if that warrants lax enforcement of law, has not made things any better. The process of reforms had picked up after 2014.

In addition to amending the Drugs & Cosmetics Rules, 1945, framing of Medical Devices Rules, 2017 and New Drugs and Clinical Trial Rules, 2019, the drafts of other rules had also been prepared for managing other aspects of drug regulation. The strengthening of existing and the proposed setting up of new drug control laboratories was a good beginning. However, in many cases, the infrastructure created could not be utilized due to non-availability of required resources. The new rules have brought a lot of clarity in regulation of medical devices, new drugs and clinical trials. Some of the structured training programs that were started during 2015-17 for drug regulators from the Centre and states have since been stopped and no long-term training and development plan has been put in place.

The vision of political leadership, be it the ruling party or the opposition, has remained confined to winning the next round of electoral battles. With the regularity of elections to one or the other legislative body or local authorities, there is hardly any dull moment. The political discourse has reached its nadir and the energy of political leaders is spent on scoring brownie points, propagating divisive or populist agenda or digging dirt from the past. The bureaucracy, especially the higher management, is too busy in furthering its own interests, and the role of assisting the political leadership to stay on course has been largely abandoned.

In the process, India continues to perform far worse than countries that began their developmental journey roughly at the same time as India did. Certainly, the authorities were not up to the challenge and their thought processes were severely constrained. The authorities have continued to refuse to dream big and most of the policies and plans were woven around the theme of scarcity, incremental changes and were based on a blurred vision. China, Japan, South Korea, Taiwan and even other emerging economies of Asia have demonstrated that better planning and implementation can make all the difference.

The crisis of accountability of the structures reflects systemic failure. Cosmetic changes continue to be made to showcase substantial improvements in areas such as those pertaining to ease of doing business. The ground reality, however remains that things have not seen any massive improvement except in some states.

The bureaucratic structures, including the technical manpower, are potent instrumentalities of the state and these can deliver efficiently. Within organizations, continuity of the leadership and implementation teams is necessary for ensuring both delivery and accountability. It is essential to repose faith in officials and hold them accountable for deficiency in delivery. Post 2014, the lateral shifting of senior officials has been far too frequent to hold anyone accountable for the shortfalls in outcomes. Further, the stifling of the structures by denying required resources, personnel, money and material to handle operations entrusted to them efficiently, is an art that has been perfected. It makes no sense to set up new organizations when the existing ones are struggling. Also, the non-utilization of facilities for want of human resources or equipment, or both only erodes the credibility of the system.

The reforms of the drug regulatory structures and adherence to total quality management at every level in each medical product manufacturing unit can wait no longer, and any further delay would be to India's disadvantage. It requires no genius to discern that the reputational damage has undermined pharmaceutical exports and if corrective steps are not taken now, the sector's export earnings could also be severely dented in the not-too distant a future. Mismanagement of the sector over decades has also created powerful, vested and deeply entrenched interest groups and these, sometimes, pose a serious threat to India's reputation in the medical products sector.

There is a need for focusing on innovation. This will entail accelerating the approvals by making the regulatory pathways and processes shorter through a single window clearance mechanism and protection of intellectual property rights; incentivizing R&D through schemes such as restructured PLI, risk sharing and tax exemption; and collaboration between the public and private players to gainfully utilize the spare facility, wherever it exists.

The PLI schemes as these are currently structured may not be able to fully sub-serve the objectives of making India competitive globally; attracting investment; ensuring efficiencies; and driving innovations in the cutting edge technologies. However, what is important is that the missing elements can be included after further consultations with the stakeholders and the government appears to be alive to this situation as demonstrated by changes in PLI 2.0 for the pharmaceutical sector.

India cannot turn a blind eye to the fact that already a large number of new players are waiting in the wings to grab the opportunity and seek to knock the Indian pharmaceutical sector out of the reckoning. Only the strictest adherence to quality and economies of scale can lead to cost cutting and help in realizing the potential of the Indian industry. As of now, none of the prospective competitors can match India both in quality and quantity fronts at the same time, and that will be India's strength. It needs to be remembered that tolerance of inefficiencies and quality compromises could make the most promising Indian sector an orphan.

The Indian industry can succeed by taking bold steps and engaging in serious introspection. The COVID-19 crisis has demonstrated that Indian Industry has the required resilience. At the same time, it has highlighted many chinks, including in terms of India's import dependence for raw materials for the production of vaccines and drugs and its failure to honor international commitments. Post the onset of the COVID-19 pandemic, the global architecture has already been signaling a move away from China-centric manufacturing. This offers a unique, a never-before second opportunity for India to scale up. However, it will require a lot of work in terms of developing, adopting and adapting standards/practices and establishing the required systems for quality assurance.

Developments post the onset of COVID-19 show that the world is ready to acknowledge it when India moves. UN Secretary-General Antonio Guterres summed up the contribution of India's pharmaceutical sector in a news conference on 29.12.2020, when he described India as the pharmaceutical powerhouse and an important element in the democratization of access to medicines all over the world. Referring to vaccine production, UN Secretary-General had stated that the production capacity of India is one of the best assets the world has, and it must be fully used. The chinks that have been noticed, if addressed, can help in realizing the India dream.

India needs to play a much bigger role in the global healthcare delivery and move beyond just being the manufacturer of generic medicines and expand the bouquet of services that it could offer. The failure of many countries to respond efficiently to the COVID-19 pandemic, including some well-off countries, and the inability of many others to take care of everyone who needed such care, also throws up new opportunities in the field of human healthcare. Demographic dividend is a potential and the benefit will accrue only if it can be channelized while it is available.

For realizing the potential of Indian industry, directionless growth of the pharmaceuticals and medical devices industry has to be replaced by a well-calibrated action plan. It should not require one more pandemic to reform the structures and create the required ecosystem for these sectors to deliver. The successful transition of the Indian industry to a world-class pharmaceutical and medical devices manufacturing hub will, besides intent, require a robust regulatory structure, consistency in policies, including with regard to incentives for manufacturing and research & development, handholding of industry and rendering assistance for managing crisis and improved information dissemination. Inadequate thrust on research & development and the failure of public facilities/laboratories and other scientific departments/institutions to contribute to any significant extent in drug development and discovery also needs to be reversed.

Indian participation in clinical research and clinical trials has also been limited and disproportionately lower than what should be legitimately expected from a country of India's size, stature and ethnic diversity. The future of medicines is biologicals/biopharmaceuticals. Therefore, drug discovery has to move to new areas like biopharmaceuticals, stem cells, regenerative medicines and other non-conventional therapies that are fast emerging as more effective therapeutic solutions. It will be necessary to address the reasons that drive the pre-clinical research and clinical trials away from the country and initiate necessary remedial measures.

In the light of the foregoing, to say that all is fine with the Indian medical products sector would apparently be false. The Indian pharmaceutical and, to some extent, medical devices industry are afflicted on account of a whole lot of problems. The medical products industry may still not be in the ICU but it definitely is ailing and needs urgent intervention to stop further deterioration. It needs to be recognized that with plenty of cheap labor and a number of factories, making generic drugs is no big deal. It is the quality of the product that can make Indian generics useful and marketable. With the application of the latest technology and artificial intelligence, the possibility of fully automated generic drug factories could soon be a reality. The Indian pharmaceutical and medtech industry can survive only by putting the quality first.

The impact of disruptive technologies on healthcare delivery is set to irreversibly alter the patient-doctor relationships in future. Eric Topol, in his book[3] *provides a glimpse of the kind of* power that the patient has started wielding with the new age technologies that includes smart-phones and a variety of biosensors. These shift the control of healthcare away from the doctor, the government and others. Indian healthcare sector needs to be prepared for not only manufacturing the state-of-the-art medical products but also adopt the new technology for the benefit of the human beings. This could go a long way in India moving towards the ultimate destination for healthcare for the globe as a whole.

While the task at hand might appear to be daunting, India has the required capacity and the resilience to realize its true potential. For this, there has to be a conscious strategy to move away from the current state

---

[3.] 'The Patient Will See You Now: The Future of Medicine is in Your Hands'

of affairs to a new trajectory that can only take the Indian industry to the top of the pyramid. It needs to be remembered that the choice is to climb and reach the summit irrespective of the hurdles, or slide down the hill and be decimated. Just hoping for it to happen on its own would be a sure shot for disaster, and doing it, on the other hand, is not impossible. In the competitive world that we are living in, the price of delay could be disastrous.

Fortunately, the winds of change are blowing. Many pharmaceutical manufacturers and the majority of medical device manufacturers realize that there is no point in continuing with the *status quo* and that the Indian medical product manufacturers need to adhere to the highest standard of quality in sync with the best in the world. Many of them are ready to take bold and strategic moves into uncharted territories, including developing technology platforms, foraying into new areas such as biopharmaceuticals, biosimilars and next-gen APIs like ionic liquids, etc.,[4] as well as expanding exports to non-traditional markets. For this, the unqualified support of the governmental authorities will be needed.

The industry also recognizes the need to protect its position through adoption of new-age digital and advanced analytics techniques to drive newer efficiencies across front-end and back-end operations.[5] Many in the industry are clear that it will be no longer feasible to continue to market or export not of standard quality products, and improving the quality of products can be deferred no longer.

As far as the government is concerned, the pharmaceutical and medical device sectors were chosen for focused attention under the 'Make in India' program after the 2014 elections by Modi government. In the first five years of Narendra Modi's tenure as the Prime Minister of India, while the intent was always there, the government failed to provide any

---

[4.] Ionic liquids are compounds composed completely of ions with melting point below 100 °C. These became a major scientific area almost one century after the discovery of first such compound. These have innovative applications in drug synthesis and drug delivery systems.

[5.] https://www.ipa-india.org/wp-content/uploads/2020/10/indian-pharmaceutical-industry-way-forward.pdf

major impetus for the transition. The only significant achievements of the first tenure of the Modi government were the notification of the Medical Devices Rules, 2017, some improvements in the clinical trials environment, conceptualization and execution of the Andhra Pradesh Medtech Zone and the good work done for evolving standards for medical devices. The exponential growth of the sector, leading to scaling of new heights visualized under the 'Make in India' program, however, remained a pipe dream.

The second tenure of the Modi government has witnessed some more positive steps for ushering in policy-level changes to improve the ecosystem. The Production Linked Incentive schemes for pharmaceuticals, bulk drugs and medical devices, and development of medical devices are decisions in the right direction; however, these could have been structured better had meaningful, free and frank discussion been held with the stakeholders. The decision-making processes have also improved, as evidenced by faster approvals under the PLI schemes. However, the vision is still not broad enough to raise India to be a major global player. The implementation of these schemes will also need to be watched carefully as the credentials of the government in such matters are suspect. The other areas, including legal and organizational overhaul, the regulation of medical products, and pharmaceutical and medtech education also need urgent corrective action. It will be instructive to study why the NIPERs could not succeed just like the IITs and IIMs did.

To conclude, it would not be wrong to say that the Indian medical products sector has the opportunity to be at the forefront of innovation by internalizing the technological disruptions and accelerating change. Rather than being content with the spasmodic reforms that move two steps forward and one and a half step backward, the reform process has to gather the speed, scale and substance of a Tsunami that encourages entrepreneurship and innovation.

India has all that it requires to leapfrog to the top league of medical products manufacturing countries. What needs to be done is fixing a few nuts and bolts here and there in accordance with a well-thought out multipronged strategy. When it comes to doing it, India can do it. Many more new doors will open for the Indian healthcare industry if the country can integrate and internalize quality in all processes of manufacturing and handling medical products. Further, making public health- related R&D a priority will ensure better health outcomes globally and generate additional employment opportunities. The success of the pharmaceutical and medical devices sectors could catapult India to become the ultimate destination for healthcare facilities for people from across countries and continents.

A journey of a thousand miles certainly begins with a single step; the medical products sector will, however, not be able to manage with baby steps. It will have to be a giant leap that provides enough thrust to escape the prevalent inertia. An enterprising and a great country with high aspirations cannot be held back for long by those who refuse to see beyond the next elections; or self-promoting bureaucracy; or even by some desperate elements in the industry whose entire interest lies in minting profit, even if these be at the cost of public health. *Alia iacta est* or the die is cast, India does not have much of a choice; the medical products sector has to transition and transition fast for the sake of humanity, and it cannot afford to fail. One can do no better than to wrap up in the words of the former President of India, Dr. APJ Abdul Kalam that we should not give up and we should not allow the problem to defeat us.

APPENDIX

REBOOTING MEDICAL PRODUCTS SECTOR

THE LEGAL AND ADMINISTRIVE ARCHITECTURE

1. Amend Schedule Seven of the Constitution of India to place public health in the Concurrent list and Drugs and Medical devices in the Union list

2. Undertake consultations with all concerned – nationally and internationally – for evolving a new legislative framework, including a new law and new rules for regulating the pharmaceutical and medtech sectors. This exercise can be completed in a period of around two years. This would entail replacement of the archaic pre-independence Drugs & Cosmetics Act, 1940 by a new central law that comprehensively covers regulation of manufacturing, sale and marketing of Drugs; Cosmetics; New Drug & Clinical Trials; Medical Devices; and regulation of advertisements relating to medical products in different sections. The new law should be in conformity with the best international practices and be a model for others to emulate.

3. Amend all other related laws to bring them in conformity with the proposed legal framework. A single amending legislation will be desirable for ensuring uniformity.

4. Replace the existing fragmented structures under the Centre and the states by a single world-class statutory and autonomous regulator for medical products for the country as a whole. India will do better with 'One nation, one law and one regulator for medical products', rather than three dozen-plus drug regulators. In the process, the state drug regulators will get merged with the central regulator. The new authority can be designated as the National Medical Products Regulatory Authority (NMPRA).

5. NMPRA cannot be a Subordinate Office of the DGHS, which itself is an Attached Office of the MoHFW. It may be restructured as a statutory and autonomous authority answerable to the MoHFW only for purposes of accountability to the Parliament and discharge of other legal formalities. It should have full autonomy in operational matters.

6. The Governing Body of the NMPRA should comprise Health Secretary; Secretary, Department of Health Research; Secretary, Department of Biotechnology; Director General, Health Services, Financial Adviser in the Ministry; Drugs Controller General and a representative each from the associations of pharmaceutical industry, medical devices industry and consumer/patient care organizations. Joint Secretary (R) in the MoHFW can be the Member Secretary. The Governing body should only look into policy-related issues and not the day-to-day administration.

7. Drugs Controller General may be nominated as the chief executive of NMPRA and authorized to dispose of regular business. He may be given the rank and status of Special Secretary to the Government of India.

8. NMPRA may be organized on functional lines, with each vertical disposing of the major part of its business at its own level and only very complex cases being put up to the DCG(I). The verticals can be on the lines suggested in the report of the Satyananda Mishra Committee in 2015. The law should authorize the government to add to or reduce the number of verticals.

9. Separate verticals may be headed by experts in the relevant fields in grades equivalent to the Joint Secretary to the Government of India. The verticals to be created could be one each for (i) Drugs; (ii) Biologicals, Stem Cells and other emerging areas; (iii) Medical Devices; (iv) Quality Control, Drug Testing and Analysis; (v) Ayush; (vi) Cosmetics and (vi) Surveillance and Prosecution. Each vertical should have a number of specialists in the relevant disciplines to steer the work.

10. The surveillance and prosecution work should be managed centrally and the entire database should be available in user-friendly software. Prosecutions should not depend on the whims and fancies of Drug Inspectors. The authority for initiating prosecution should be exercised centrally after due approvals by the authorities to be specified for the purpose. Timelines will need to be fixed for filing cases and responsibility fixed for any unusual delay. A set of qualified legal practitioners may assist in the prosecution.

11. The terms/words used in the Act may be defined with clarity and to the extent feasible; the terms already defined in the Medical Devices Rules, 2017 and New Drugs & Clinical Trial Rules, 2019 may be used as such. Effort should be to incorporate internationally accepted terminology.

12. The transgressions and offenses may be clearly segregated, with only financial penalties for transgressions that do not have *mens rea* associated with it. In other words, transgressions without mens rea may be decriminalized.

13. The penalties/punishment for manufacturing, import and sale or marketing of substandard drugs and medical devices may be rationalized. The penalty/punishment may be staggered, keeping in view the gravity of the offense. The penalty should be in proportion to the transgression.

14. Separate provisions may be made for regulating medical devices in conformity with GHTF framework.

15. Completely distinct courts be established in each district or for a group of districts for trial of medical products-related offenses, and timelines may be stipulated for disposal of cases by such courts. Appeals from the decisions of such courts may lie only to the High Court.

16. The powers of Inspectors may be clearly specified and the powers of other authorities may also be specified in the proposed legislation. It would be necessary to curb arbitrariness in their actions.

17. The autonomy of the regulator should extend to removing its dependence on the government for resources, whether financial or human. This can be done by rationalizing the fee structure. An

assessment undertaken in 2016 by the MoHFW indicated that it was feasible over a period of ten years.

18. Bridge the mismatch between infrastructure, human resources and equipment in all organizations working in the field of drugs

19. A separate high-powered appellate mechanism may be set up to examine appeals and take a final decision in a time-bound manner in all cases where a manufacturer wants to file an appeal against the decisions of the regulator.

20. Clear, transparent and objective provisions may be made for compounding cases. Details of all cases compounded may be placed in the public domain with reasoned order.

21. Highest levels of transparency may be ensured to minimize the scope for colorful exercise of discretion by officials. In all cases where discretion has been exercised one way or the other, a reasoned order will be required to be issued and it should be subject to periodic audit by a pre-specified agency.

22. Set up a robust mechanism for vigilance to curb corruption, bribery and other malpractices

23. The procedure for different kinds of inspections be made in the regulations to be framed under the law. Officials trained in GMP and GLP may only be deputed for inspections, and provision be made for placing the findings of the inspections in the public domain.

24. Provisions may be added to the Act for continuous education and learning of regulators and their continuation in certain roles may be subject to qualifying examination at regular intervals of time.

25. Re-equip existing Drug Testing Laboratories in each state, set up new laboratories and increase the picking up and testing of samples four-fold.

26. Provisions may be made for audit of all the decisions taken by regulatory authorities by external auditors, some of whom could be the retired and experienced regulators from stringent regulatory structures.

27. NMPRA may be authorized to suspend or cancel the licenses issued for manufacturing and for sale of medical products for reasons to

be recorded in writing. Such order will be subject to review by the competent authority specified in the Act.

28. Certifying bodies may be set up for reducing the regulatory burden of NMPRA and appropriate mechanisms be made for ensuring that such bodies are fully equipped to handle the work.

29. The certification undertaken by certification bodies approved by the CDSCO under ICMED scheme may be accepted for regulatory purposes.

HUMAN RESOURCES MANAGEMENT

30. Development and training of professionals for regulation of medical products is critical for the growth of the pharmaceutical and medtech sectors because any further growth of the two would be feasible only if the quality of the product can be ensured and the market for Indian products expanded to include new therapies. That will be possible only if regulatory structures have competent and efficient human resources.

31. Increase the strength of regulatory and laboratory officials, with the total number of personnel to be pegged at around 20,000 for the country as a whole. Officials with specialization in different areas may be recruited.

32. Revise all recruitment rules and make arrangements for expeditious filling up of all vacancies. No post should be allowed to remain vacant for more than six months and if necessary, to begin with, the vacancies be filled up through contractual appointments pending regular recruitment in a staggered manner.

33. Set up a world-class training academy for drug regulators and officials for medical products regulation, testing and analysis, for which the trainers may be drawn from within the country and abroad. Trainers from outside the government may be taken for fixed tenures of up to five years on market-driven salaries.

34. The training academy should also have paid courses for professionals from medical products industry. It should start courses for industry

professionals, and for certain roles in the industry, it may be made mandatory to have acquired proficiency in the specified areas.

35. Targeted training and development activities be planned after assessing the required competencies and skill sets at different levels.

36. Cultural shifts and changes in attitude, practices and behavior of individuals, groups and organizations may be included in all training programs.

37. The required pool of competent trainers may be created within the world-class training academy for imparting knowledge about Good Manufacturing Practices, Good Clinical Practices, Good Laboratory Practices, Good Storage and Distribution Practices, and other relevant aspects to regulators and industry professionals on payment.

38. Retrain and redeploy all officials to ensure that they are in a position to render useful services. Offer voluntary cessation scheme to those who are found to be not fit for retention after assessment.

39. To avoid unnecessary litigation, bring out recruitment rules for all posts in a time-bound manner, keeping in view the competencies required.

40. Open all drug testing laboratories for paid internship to students in relevant disciplines for a period of three to six months

41. Training may include both regulatory and laboratory functions. Both sets of officials should be trained in laboratory as well as regulatory practices. Further, all officials recruited up to the level of Drug Inspectors should work in laboratories for at least three years. The working in the laboratory may be made mandatory for promotion to the grade of Assistant Drug Controllers.

42. Pending creation of the posts and hiring of the required talent on regular basis, specialists be drawn from alternate sources, including from amongst PIOs for important positions.

43. The National Institute of Biologicals should set up a separate Wing for undertaking activities that could help in providing necessary guidance to industry to overcome any difficulties that the industry working in the area of biologicals and IVDs may face. It should become the

go-to place for the industry for assistance and guidance in case of all biologicals.

44. The Indian Pharmacopoeia Commission should commence training programs for industry professionals and it should be mandated to impart guidance on quality control, testing and analysis to industry professionals.

45. The Indian Pharmacopoeia Commission should also open up its facilities for internships and training to more students from different universities/institutions to provide exposure to them to the state-of-the-art facilities and equip them to be industry-ready by acting as a finishing school.

46. The Post marketing surveillance activities may be suitably stepped up. The training programs in the field of pharmacovigilance, materiovigilance, haemovigilance and AEFI may be stepped up by the respective institutions and these be opened up for professionals from the industry. Online and distance-mode courses may also be started for continuous up gradation of the skill sets by tying up with SWYAM or other similar programs.

REVAMP DECISION-MAKING PROCESSES

47. Strengthen field-level implementation and do not allow excuses for non-delivery of the agreed deliverables and hold the structures accountable

48. Fix timelines for decision making and set up a mechanism for quality audit of decisions made, including by subject experts/advisory/other committees, and make the results public. Wherever feasible, engage international experts in the field for undertaking quality audit. Such audit should not be for fault finding but for identifying deficiencies and initiating necessary corrective action.

49. In the case of new drug approvals, ensure parallel processing to reduce time required for according approvals. Multiple clearances required

from the CDSCO, GEAC and RCGM or any other authority should be made online and given within the timelines fixed for each category.

50. Pre-submission facilitation should be structured within the CDSCO on payment basis for all kinds of clearances.

51. The meetings of the Subject Expert Committees need to be facilitated through *SUGAM* or any other suitable mechanism, obviating the need for physical meetings.

52. The huge gaps in the quality of information currently available with multiple regulatory agencies regarding drug regulation may be bridged through various measures, including the facility to send automated notices on drug recall to distributors and retailers.

53. Leverage technology to make the process of obtaining licenses easier for clients.

54. The approval process for new medical products should be automated to the extent feasible, and each vertical should have in-house experts in the relevant fields who could work full-time post-retirement from the government. In addition to that, panels of experts in relevant specialties could be prepared for specific work.

55. Ensure inspection of all manufacturing facilities at least once in a year. The inspections should be coordinated and where regulators of importing countries intend to inspect the manufacturing facilities, arrangements may be made for joint inspection to minimize the dislocation of normal working of manufacturing units.

56. No manufacturing facility having critical deficiencies may be allowed to remain operational till the deficiency is removed.

57. Sharing of information with the surveillance and vigilance wing of the CDSCO for all field officials, including the purpose of the visit of any regulatory official to manufacturing facilities and findings thereof, be made mandatory.

58. At least one inspection of the retail and wholesale marketing/sales facilities/outfits be undertaken each year.

59. The governmental stores and pharmacies may be targeted for additional quality checks and inspections in view of the larger NSQ drugs noticed in government supply chain.

60. Representatives of civil society organizations selected through a transparent process be associated in all inspections.

RAMP UP MANUFACTURING

61. Take decisive steps to ensure that the production linked schemes for pharmaceuticals, medical devices, bulk drug parks and medical devices parks succeed, and the incentives may be revisited if considered expedient for better results.

62. Set up a task force to identify critical areas that hold up the utilization of full manufacturing capacity, especially with regard to the availability of raw materials, as was noticed in case of manufacture of vaccines for handling the COVID-19 pandemic

63. Ensure consistency in the business environment and do not alter the same retrospectively, leading to genuine profit not being earned by industry

64. Revisit the scheme for price fixation of drugs and medical devices, thus allowing prices to be remunerative. This will reduce the temptation to compromise on quality.

65. Revisit the PMBJP as it is based on defective premises and could cause unwarranted damage to both the patients and the industry

66. Rationalize customs duty on drugs and medical devices. It should be raised to the maximum permissible limit under the WTO arrangements to incentivize domestic manufacturing. The increase can be given effect to in a staggered manner.

67. Rationalize GST and custom duty on drugs and medical devices

68. Liberalize FDI with cap on maximum holding by foreign entities and minimum Indian shareholding.

69. Provide support for patent filing to make the process easier; refund the foreign trademark registration fee.

70. Bridge the gap between the intention and the actual delivery at the ground level by streamlining implementation

71. Labeling requirements for indicating the country of origin may be insisted upon.

72. The validity of Free Sale Certificate may be suitably enhanced.

QUALITY IMPROVEMENT

73. The entire data, starting with procurement of API/KSM/DI, manufacturing, distribution, storage, dispensing and recall of medicines, be digitalized to ensure non-introduction of spurious products in the supply chain. The process will help in tracking and tracing each strip/vial of medicine from manufacturer to the patient and help in recall and disposal of defective medicines. The concept note on regulation of e-pharmacies placed in the public domain in 2016 by the MoHFW had visualized such a system. The same can be used as the template for evolving the system.

74. Clamp down on non-licensed manufacturers of medical products and ensure all such units are closed and criminal proceedings initiated against the owners of such units.

75. The manufacturing units that are not meeting the GMP requirements or manufacture products without establishing therapeutic equivalence where it is considered necessary or have not done stability testing, may be ordered to be closed down.

76. A mechanism be established for expeditious review of the medicines that have been approved in the past to reassess their therapeutic utility in view of the latest developments in the field of medical sciences. The medical products that are not rational any more, be weeded out.

77. Resume inspection of API/KSM/DI manufacturing sites from where imports will be allowed and make it at least an annual inspection. No imports be allowed from the manufacturers that have not been inspected in that particular year. The fee for such inspection be kept at a higher level.

78. Incentivize integrity programs for ensuring compliances and provide all possible support to the industry for migrating to best-quality manufacturing of medical products at the lowest cost. The choice to shut down be given to those who cannot upgrade to the acceptable level of quality.

79. Robust data reliability systems be put in place by leveraging technology, upgrade systems and capabilities in investigations; strengthen management systems for quality, even with increasing operational complexity.

80. Enforce manufacturers to embed quality into product design and build a culture of quality across organizations.

81. Establish synergy between the CDSCO and other standard setting bodies and develop as many standards as possible at the earliest.

UPGRADE THE IT INFRASTRUCTURE

82. Upscale the IT infrastructure including *SUGAM* appropriately to facilitate all transactions and fix the glitches that still remain unresolved. *SUGAM* may be further strengthened to provide for online clearance by concerned authority on the pattern of the Project Monitoring System established initially in the Cabinet Secretariat, and cases where approval or rejection is not communicated within the time-limit, should lead to responsibility being fixed.

83. *XLN* software be integrated with *SUGAM*, and eventually all activities be made online.

84. Drug Authentication and Verification Application (DAVA) of the Department of Commerce, Government of India, be upgraded and integrated with *SUGAM*. It may be made mandatory for all manufacturers to operate the DAVA within a year. Its integration with quality assurance mechanism discussed in the context of e-pharmacies above may be explored.

ENHANCE COLLABORATION

85. The facilities available in the ICMR, CSIR and DBT institutions may be opened up to companies interested in undertaking research in a particular area on payment basis.

86. Make it mandatory for each government laboratory to tie up at least for research in one particular area with the private sector for developing newer technologies. Let each laboratory publicize what it can offer to the private sector and at what cost.

87. Translation of basic research to end-products for use in real life be taken up on a mission mode

88. India should join PIC/S and aim at complete harmonization of regulatory practices with the best global practices. This would be necessary as expectations of regulatory organizations around the world have increased and a number of Indian companies are manufacturing and supplying medicines to well-regulated markets.

89. Indian manufacturing facilities are inspected by regulators from every country that buys Indian medicines. Amongst others, these include the USA, the UK, Germany, South Korea, Japan and Brazil. As a result, Indian pharmaceutical companies catering to foreign markets have strengthened their processes, improved automation, operating procedures and quality management systems. Progressively, introduce similar inspection of manufacturers not catering to foreign markets on an experimental basis by some of these regulators. A reciprocal arrangement for this could be worked out with some of the leading regulatory authorities.

90. Work towards interoperability between the regulators of importing countries and Indian regulators through increased interaction, joining each other's training programs and joint inspections

91. The National Academy for Drug Regulators may conduct paid courses for inspectors from the importing countries to ensure that they are able to function effectively while conducting inspection of the Indian manufacturing units. This will empower them to better understand Indian culture, ethos and manufacturing practices.

CLINICAL TRIALS AND RESEARCH & DEVELOPMENT

92. Reset the priority from being the producer of 'low-cost' generics to high-quality pharmaceuticals/biopharmaceuticals and make India a hub for clinical research and trials. The government/public institutions will have to play a leading role in this.

93. Allow decisions to relax or remove restrictions on import/export of Genetically Modified Organisms/clones/large and other animals for use by the organizations concerned and a speaking note should be issued by the agency concerned in such cases to allow for audit of the decisions at a later stage. The note should be shared with the regulatory authorities concerned on a real-time basis.

94. The Institutional Animal Ethics Committee and Institutional Bio-safety Committee with respect to toxicology studies of biologically derived products be strengthened and only properly qualified persons be appointed on these committees.

95. The pool for undertaking toxicological studies should also be expanded and the Indian Institute of Toxicology Research could be given the target for developing necessary manpower.

96. Procedures for use of animals in research & development activities may be streamlined and timelines/thresholds laid down for decision making. The highly restrictive clearance mechanism may be replaced by a pragmatic approach.

97. Wherever necessary, take up R&D of new products in collaboration with leading scientific institutions within the country and in developed countries, and augment the quality of existing products substantially.

98. Nurture Indian companies to be ethical and make them understand that they can expand and continue to meet the growing demand for medicines across the world only by complying with the regulatory and quality requirements

99. On an experimental basis, handover the management of a few laboratories of the CSIR and ICMR to the best experts from across the globe. Tap PIO/NRI resources for this. The arrangement should be at

least for a period of ten years and their progress should be monitored/ reviewed at pre-decided periodicity.

UTILIZATION OF PUBLIC SECTOR VACCINE FACILITIES

100. Convert the Central Research Institute (CRI), Kasauli into an Institute of National of Importance for teaching, training and research in the field of vaccinology and related areas, and make it into an autonomous body on the pattern of IITs and, where feasible, tie-ups with reputed international institutions

101. Make concrete plans for utilization of manufacturing capacities at CRI, Kasauli, the Pasteur Institute of India, Coonoor, the BCG Vaccine Laboratory, Chennai and HLL Biotech Ltd. (HBL), a recent state-of-the-art WHO-pre-qualified facility at Chengalpattu, Chennai; if necessary, by partnering with the private sector. International collaboration may also be explored.

102. Feasibility of other state-run utilities partnering with private sector manufactures may also be explored.

103. Make a comprehensive plan of action for augmentation of innovations and R&D in India through partnership between the public and private sectors

104. Provide hands-on support to industry by making the public facilities available for research, development, testing, analysis and imparting training to professionals.

105. Strengthen post marketing surveillance of drugs; medical devices; blood transfusions and AEFI. Establish robust institutional arrangements for capturing and analyzing data.

PRODUCTION LINKED INCENTIVE SCHEMES

106. A PLI scheme may be introduced for augmenting research and developmental activities by the private sector. Partnership with institutions in the public sector may be incentivized.

107. Ensure continuity of the schemes over a longer period of time with such modifications as may be necessary to attract investors and quality manufacturers. The PLI schemes for bulk drug parks, medical device parks and pharmaceuticals may be further honed in consultations with the stakeholders.

108. Scale up all the PLI schemes as these are still not ambitious enough for a country of India's size and potential.

109. Expeditiously review all the schemes and come out with a modified mega plan to make India the global medical devices manufacturing hub.

110. Come out with a PLI scheme for chemical industry for ensuring availability of the raw materials and solvents, etc., for APIs/formulations.

111. Encourage setting up pharmaceutical machine manufacturing facilities in India to lower fixed costs, enable savings in forex and reduce time to set up additional facilities. Include this within the ambit of PLI.

112. Bolster the logistics infrastructure for connecting the key pharmaceutical hubs in the country to facilitate quick and cost-efficient movement of goods, including cold chain facilities

113. Address the challenge of proper storage and transportation of medical products and also evolve a scheme for up gradation of these facilities.

114. All PLI schemes should move from import substitution to building globally competitive Indian multinationals.

FINE-TUNING PROCUREMENT PROCESSES

115. Fine-tune the government procurement processes to ensure that medical products of dubious quality are not procured. For this, elaborate guidelines may be firmed up to ensure uniformity across the board.

116. In case of medicines, procurements may be restricted to the manufacturers who have complied with the required processes and where the manufacturing facility is fully GMP-compliant.

117. In case of medical devices, it may be ensured that the second-hand refurbished equipment is not allowed to be imported into the country in the name of cost-effective solutions.

118. A high-level committee may be set up to lay down the standards that are to be followed in case of different medical devices and equipment and beyond that, no discretion may be permitted to any governmental agency procuring them. The feasibility of establishing synergy between the CDSCO, QCI and BIS for standard setting may be explored.

119. Sterile devices may not be permitted to be used more than once. Single use medical devices may not be allowed to be used more than once.

JUDICIAL INTERVENTION IN MATTERS OF SCIENCE

120. The Supreme Court of India may lay down clear and mandatory guidelines for the High Courts to follow in cases impacting human and animal health. This would be necessary to prevent breaching the boundaries through judicial intervention in matters of public health. The procedural and technical reasons may not be allowed to play havoc with human health, and the judiciary should be sensitized to honor science- based decisions.

121. Other suggestions given in different chapters may be acted upon.

ABBREVIATIONS

ADRs	Adverse Drug Reactions
AE	Adverse event
AEFI	Adverse Event Following Immunization
AMC	Adverse Drug Reaction Monitoring Centers
API	Active Pharmaceutical Ingredient
BIS	Bureau of Indian Standards
CDSCO	Central Drugs Standard Control Organization
CRI	Central Research Institute
CSIR	Council for Scientific and Industrial Research
DBT	Department of Bio-technology
DCC	Drug Consultative Committee
DCG(I)	Drug Controller General, India
DGHS	Director General Health Services
DI	Drug Intermediates
DST	Department of Science & Technology
DTAB	Drugs Technical Advisory Board
FDCs	Fixed Dose Combinations
GCP	Good Clinical Practices
GEAC	Genetic Engineering Appraisal Committee
GMP	Good Manufacturing Practices
IPC	Indian Pharmacopoeia Commission
ICSR	Individual Case Safety Reports
HPLC	High Performance Liquid Chromatography
HvPI	Haemo-vigilance Program of India
IEC	Institutional Ethics Committee
IIM	Indian Institute of Management
IIT	Indian Institute of Technology
IPC	Indian Pharmacopoeia Commission

KSM	Key starting Materials
MAH	Marketing Authorization Holder
MEDTECH	Medical technology
MvPI	Materio-vigilance Program of India
NIB	National Institute of Biotechnology
NIPER	National Institute of Pharmaceutical Education& research
NMPRA	National Medical Products Regulatory Authority
NRA	National Regulatory Authority
NSQ	Not of Standard Quality
OSD	Officer on Special Duty
PIC/S	Pharmaceutical Inspection Co-operation Scheme
PLI	Production Linked Scheme
PMBJP	Pradhan Mantri Bhartiya Jan Aushadhi Pariyojna
PMS	Post Marketing Surveillance
PS	Private Secretary
PSUR	Periodic safety Update Report
PvPI	Pharmacovigilance Programme of India
QCI	Quality Council of India
RCGM	Review Committee on Genetic Manipulation
SEC	Subject Expert Committee
TRP	Television(Target) Rating Points
USFDA	United States Food and Drug Administration
UN	United Nations
WHO	World Health Organization

www.ingramcontent.com/pod-product-compliance
Lightning Source LLC
Chambersburg PA
CBHW02085818O526
45163CB00007B/2548